Keeping It Off

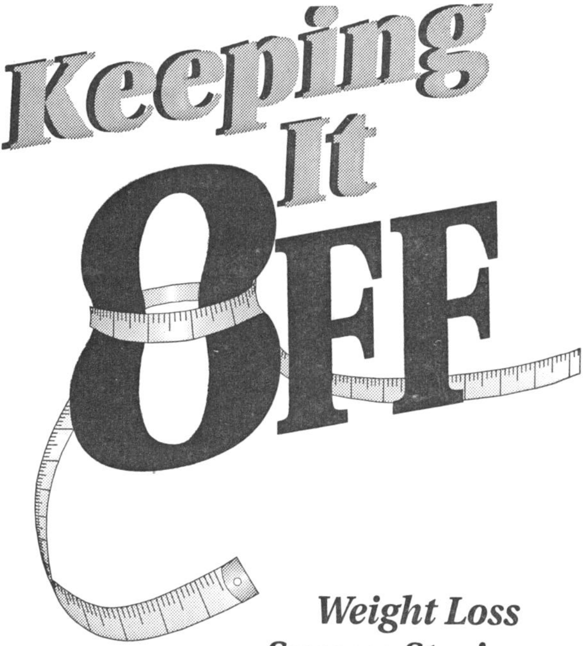

Weight Loss Success Stories from those who did it!

By Barbara Stitt, Ph.D.
& Melissa Luedtke

Keeping It Off!

Published by Natural Press
P.O. Box 730
Manitowoc, Wisconsin 54221

Disclaimer: All information in this book is for informational purposes only. None of the suggestions are intended to diagnose, prevent, or treat a disease. It is suggested that anyone wishing to make use of this information consult the relevant resources and confer with a medical professional with expertise in this area.

Printed in the United States of America

ISBN 978-0-939956-02-9

Dedication

*To all of the people who have struggled
to take it off and keep it off.*

Table Of Contents

Becoming "Food Abstinent"
from Bernice ____________ *page* 11

"Can't Eat Just One" Syndrome ____________ *page* 17

Not Just A "Diet" But A "Lifestyle"
from Kim ____________ *page* 21

Why Diets Don't Work ____________ *page* 23

Fiber
from Andy ____________ *page* 25

Divide Your Plate
from Susan ____________ *page* 29

Quality
from Andrew ____________ *page* 31

Calories And Serving Sizes
from Jackie ____________ *page* 33

A Few Helpful Hints
from Julie ____________ *page* 37

The Lean Plate Club:
Supersize That Salad ____________ *page* 39

Sugarbusters
from Nancy ____________ *page* 43

Trigger Point
from Jessica ____________ *page* 45

Size 4 Equals Size 0 ____________ *page* 49

Why Diets Don't Work ____________ *page* 23

Children At Risk _______________ *page* 53

Answers _______________ *page* 57

Sweet Tooth
from Nancy _______________ *page* 59

Fifteen Pounds
from Rebecca _______________ *page* 63

Fast Food Nation _______________ *page* 65

Four Key Factors
from Rachel _______________ *page* 69

New Hole
from Dave _______________ *page* 75

Vitamin/Mineral Deficiency
from Alexandra _______________ *page* 77

New Study Suggests Consumers Would
Like To Eat Healthier Food _______ *page* 81

Weight Watchers
from Jean _______________ *page* 83

W.W.
from Kathi _______________ *page* 85

Lifetime Member
from Sandy _______________ *page* 87

Can You Change Your Ways? _______ *page* 89

More Weight Watchers
from Karen _______________ *page* 91

Outgrown
from Barb Killen _______________ *page* 95

The Gain Game ______ *page* 97

Outside The Box
from Grace ______ *page* 103

Inspiration
from Leah ______ *page* 107

The Okinawa Plan
from Tina ______ *page* 109

Stomach Problems
from Rachael ______ *page* 111

Foodie
from Linda ______ *page* 115

Diabetic
from Carmen ______ *page* 121

Not Again
from Katherine ______ *page* 123

The Cabbage Soup Diet ______ *page* 129

Add To Your Body ______ *page* 135

Remove From Your Body ______ *page* 139

The 20 Best, Healthiest
Fat-Burning Foods ______ *page* 143

A Final Note ______ *page* 153

INTRODUCTION

Almost any diet will help you take off unwanted pounds - however *keeping the weight off* is another story. We decided to go to the experts and see how they did it. We think the following wonderful stories will warm your heart and give you the courage to clearly *go for it.* In every loaf of Natural Ovens Bakery Breads there is a Newsletter. In that Newsletter we asked people who have taken weight off and kept it off for two or more years to share their journey with us so we could share it with you. Some wonderful people have not only shared their personal stories, they have allowed us to share their 'before & after' photos.

At the end of this booklet we have also included some tips we have learned over the past 40 years of working with health – real health – the kind that makes you want to get out of bed and enjoy life to the fullest every day. Thank you for reading "Keeping it Off" and we wish you much success in going for your own goals, attaining them and maintaining them!

Barbara Stitt
President
Natural Ovens Bakery
800-558-3535
barbara.stitt@naturalovens.com

– CHAPTER ONE –

BECOMING "FOOD ABSTINENT"

from Bernice

I started "being abstinent" approximately 4-1/2 years ago. I have maintained a weight loss of 42-1/2 lbs and I feel so much better than I have felt in many years. I had been overweight all of my life, and I was never successful at weight loss programs. Weight watchers still takes my breath away; I fear that my freedom to eat when I want to will be taken from me.

When I say I have been "abstinent", I am talking about Overeaters' Anonymous (OA), and that finally worked for me. I was ready to make this change in my life. Many other changes have preceded the changes in the way I eat. I think that the change that motivated me to eat differently was that I had started to exercise and I became aware of my heavy body weighing me down; it took a lot of effort to breathe; it took a lot of effort to move. I got out of breath easily. My ability to move freely is so very precious to me. My joints no longer hurt when I move; and I do not get out of breath so fast. Besides the obvious benefits of exercise that everyone knows about, this reason has made exercise a vital part of my program.

Overeaters' Anonymous speaks of overeating as a disease, as an addiction. It has three components, the physical, the emotional and the spiritual. I will only focus on the physical. However, I truly believe that there cannot be physical recovery from this disease without addressing the emotional and the spiritual components. I truly believe that the physical symptoms are just symptoms; they are not the root of the disease.

Natural Ovens breads and muffins and Great Granola have played a very significant role in my program of recovery. Also, our children say that Paul Stitt's book, *Beating the Food Giants*, has become our "bible" on nutrition; I have read his books religiously.

I also have to give credit where credit is due. I could not have changed my life in such a meaningful way without my husband, Bruce. He has been very supportive in so many ways...too numerous to mention. He has made many of these changes in his eating too.

I made these changes very slowly. It took me about a year to lose the weight, and as my recovery grows and changes some more, I continue to fine tune and continue to make changes. When I first started this program, the first substance that I cut out was white sugar. I had very, very painful withdrawal symptoms for about six weeks. I did a lot of deep, yoga type breathing to stay with the pain, and not reach for the cake, ice cream, etc. In OA we say one day at a time. However, I must say that my abstinence is so precious to me, and I know it was worth all that pain of letting go of white sugar. I also was told in OA that I had to be willing to go to any lengths to achieve and maintain my abstinence. My body soon learned that I wasn't going to give in, and the pain of withdrawal got less and less.

I now know that I can stay away from sugar, without that initial pain, as long as I don't take that first bite. If I risk taking this substance into my body, I may go back to where I was.

Another one of my first changes was that I stopped eating when I was full, even if half the food was still on my plate. I gave up membership in the "Clean your plate" club. I was inspired to do this by a wonderful book: *Overcoming Overeating* by Jane R. Hirschmann and Carol H. Munter. This is a lot harder to do than it sounds. Social occasions where I was surrounded by loads of delicious foods are still a challenge. There is the peer pressure to overeat; everyone else is doing it and the cook may be insulted that you are eating so little. However, I have learned that the food won't run away. Thank G-d, I am not so poor that I have to eat when food is placed in front of me. I can go home and eat when I am hungry again. It took me a while to get in touch with my body's signals that I was full, to locate the thermostat. Abraham J. Twerski, M.D. in his fabulous book, *The Thin Within You*, speaks of overeater's broken thermostats and that book was extremely helpful.

This is also difficult for other reasons. We compulsive overeaters also eat for other reasons, the emotional and spiritual emptiness. If we don't feed those hungers, we tend to overeat.

I slowly identified other "trigger" foods. These are foods that I needed to avoid because they trigger me to eat more. Dried mangoes, which I love, were the first to go. The biggest change happened around a year ago. I eliminated 90% if white flour from my diet and the urge to overeat diminished even further. Natural Ovens products then became even more important to my food plan. By the way, notice that I say that the compelling urge to overeat "diminished"; it never quite goes away.

In OA we say that this disease is cunning, baffling and powerful; I would add insidious. I want to overeat by only one bite; or only take a few extra bites. I know that if I don't pay careful attention to what I am eating, I will overeat.

You can't help but notice that I don't call it a "diet." The word diet makes me very uncomfortable. Diet means rigidity, I am not rigid in my eating; I listen to my body. Then an amazing thing happened. Food started tasting so delicious! The focus of my life was no longer the food; which was amazing in and of itself! But when I do sit down to eat, I notice the deep colors of my salads; the greens of the different kinds of salads I eat. (I love to eat salads! I make a low fat dressing that no one else in my family likes; but I enjoy.) I think that food tastes are hidden when you add sugar and white flour. I was overwhelmed by the gratefulness I feel for all the delicious foods that G-d has provided us: the fruits, fishes, and whole grains.

I also try to plan my meals around foods that I love to eat and that are good for me. For example, as I have become more conscious of what I eat, I try to buy the least processed foods and if possible, buy organic. Why subject my body to the abuse of chemicals if I don't have to?

I just want to share one last insight. On our first trip away from home, Bruce pointed out that: those who fail to plan, plan to fail. Going to any length to make our programs work means that when we travel, we will call ahead to ask what our hosts are serving and we take a lot of our own food with us. We learned that you can take a cooler on the plane with you. The security people will go through the cooler and tape it back up for you. Traveling has taught us to be assertive and to ask questions.

Bernice Chicago, IL

– CHAPTER TWO –

"CAN'T EAT JUST ONE" SYNDROME

Many of American's today are just like Bernice and fail to see that they are overeating. They are hooked on potato chips, french fries, hamburgers, candy bars and cola and have become casualties of the processed food addiction; victims of the Can't Eat Just One Syndrome. What exactly causes this syndrome and how is it leading millions of Americans to become overeaters.

The organ which controls our cravings for food is called the appestat. It is located at the base of the brain. The appestat is constantly monitoring the blood for nutrient content. Only when 51 nutrients are present at their proper levels will the individual feel entirely full and satisfied. If any one nutrient is missing, the individual feels hungry. In order for an individual to feel satisfied and healthy, all of the nutrients must be present.

Think about times when you feel full after eating at an all-you-can-eat buffet. You may feel full, but you do not feel healthy. That is the difference between overeating and eating healthy. When you overeat, you will be very full and not feel very good. Usually about 1-1/2 to 2 hours later, your body will be telling you that you are hungry again. The reason this is happening is because your body did not get enough of the essential nutrients it needs to function properly. Your appestat is sending out signals to your brain to eat again in hopes that you will fill your body with what it needs: vitamins, minerals and phyto-nutrients found in fresh fruits, vegetables and fortified whole grains. They have the nutrient level your body needs to survive. If you are consuming a healthy meal and you feel full after eating, you usually feel reenergized and good because you filled up on the proper nutrients your body was craving.

Many nasty tricks are used by the food industry to seduce you into trying their foods and then they addict you which causes you to overeat. Adding lots of fat, sugar and salt are obvious ones. They know that if they add enough fat, sugar and salt Americans will eat almost anything. The real dirty tricks that food companies use to make you overeat are more subtle and do not jump out at you when you read the label – things like "artificial flavoring". These "artificial flavorings" could be nucleic acid from chromosomes of cells, extracts of yeast cells, waste beef or worse. Rabbi Eidlitz from the Kosher Information Bureau in North Hollywood, California, reported that some ingredients with names like "natural" colors have been known to contain monkey intestines and "artificial flavors" from ground-up cats.[1]

One thing for sure, it is there to make your taste buds go crazy, so that if you eat just one bite, you are hooked and have to keep right on eating until the bag is empty. The most insidious, most misleading compounds ever added to foods have the sweetest name of all – artificial sweetener – because they are not added to make foods taste sweet, they are added to make you overeat.

1 Stitt, Paul. (1993) Beating the Food Giants. Natural Press, Manitowoc, WI.

Another dirty trick the food companies have been pulling on the American public since 1911 is hydrogenated fats. They have been selling partially hydrogenated fats (margarine and shortening) as a healthy, kosher alternative to lard, butter and other fats. You'll find margarine or shortening or partially hydrogenated vegetable fat in nearly every bread, cookie and cake sold in America. In 1992, Europe started taking hydrogenated fats out of food, but American food companies are finally starting in 2005 to reduce the rise of hydrogenated fats.

There are several ways to make foods so that you can't eat just one:

- Remove fiber, protein and other nutrients
- Add appetite stimulants to the max
  - Sugar
  - Meat extracts
  - Artificial sweeteners
  - Artificial flavors

A couple of suggestions for avoiding appetite stimulating foods that lead to overeating:

- Eat whole fresh fruits, vegetables, and fortified whole grains
- Drink water
- Eat appetite satisfying foods
  - Foods fortified with vitamins and minerals
  - Foods made with flax

As Bernice and many others have found, their weight problems are linked to over eating. It is proven that the food industry is creating food that is making people crave food more, leading them to overeat. A few suggestions that we can give to avoid overeating are:

- Exercise lightly before the meal
- Enjoy multi-course, multi-colored meals
- Savor each bite
- Sit down and eat with both hands and no TV or newspapers
- Cut your food up and eat slower
- Fully chew and thoroughly enjoy every bite of your food

– CHAPTER THREE –

NOT JUST A "DIET" BUT A "LIFESTYLE"

from Kim

The key to weight loss and improving health is all in a "lifestyle" change. Until you are ready for that, those so called "diet programs" will not be successful. Yes, you will lose weight on these "diets", but what you're actually losing is lean muscle tissue, not body fat, and lowering your metabolism so that it no longer works for you. The end result of a high percentage of people will be gaining the weight back, plus more. In order to be successful with weight loss you have to "play" with your metabolism and get it working for you again.

My story is just like everybody else. I was over 40, reaching a weight I was uncomfortable with and a size jump I didn't want to make, so I was ready to make that "lifestyle" change. I thank God everyday for introducing me to Curves and what it has to offer. Curves is a fun, fast and effective way to shape up, define muscle shape, lower body fat but not losing lean muscle tissue and to learn the best strategy of how to keep your weight off once you've reached your goal. Combining three exercise components of strength training, cardio, and a target heart rate will aid you in losing your body fat, but gain much more benefits through health.

I started with Curves as a member 3 1/2 years ago and have worked for them the past 2 years. Once you've joined their program you're hooked. (I call myself a "lifer.") I lost 25 pounds of body fat and 19 inches. Who could ask for anything simpler in our busy, hectic society! Being a busy woman myself, a 30 minute, 3 times a week workout, plus through their weight management program, learning and enjoying a new lifestyle in a way I eat, I not only have my *CURVES* back, but I have the energy and outlook on a much healthier life.

So many health issues could be avoided through healthier eating choices and exercise. I know heredity plays into these issues too, but heart disease, osteoporosis, diabetes II, arthritis, and obesity could be prevented or greatly improved through proper nutrition and exercise. I would like to extend an invitation for any women out there to visit your nearest Curves and get your life back, not just for you, but for your family too.

To your health,
Kim Grafton, WI

– CHAPTER FOUR –

WHY DIETS DON'T WORK

The traditional way of losing weight by dieting, may be successful initially, but in the long run people could end up gaining a higher body fat percentage. This happens because of the psychological effects of food restrictions.

When you go on a low calorie diet, your body thinks you are starving and it starts storing fat by slowing down the metabolism. Even when the diet regime is discontinued, the metabolism is still slow and inefficient and as a result weight is gained even faster. Low calorie diets also cause you to lose muscle and water in large amounts. Besides, starving yourself may also result in decreased ability to concentrate, increase in anxiety levels, and tendency to increased alcohol consumption.

The key to healthy eating is to focus on good nutritious foods, foods of substance, and do some physical activity regularly. By exercising to the point of sweating and reducing fat supporting calories, you stand a much better chance of maintaining a healthy body. Some of the ways to nourish yourself are as follows:

- Choose nourishing foods, emphasize on garlic, onions, spinach, strawberries, beans, broccoli, carrots, sweet potatoes, soy and citrus fruits, oatmeal, whole grain breads, tomatoes, cantaloupe, and brown rice.
- Enjoy your eating, eat slowly and feel the taste of all foods.

- Listen to your body, eat when you are hungry and stop when you are full.
- Even while dieting, keep some room for your favorite foods. Eat them in small portions.
- Educate yourself about your nutritional needs.

Instead of going on a diet, choose to alter your eating habits in a way that will not affect the rest of your daily events, compromise your health, or cause you to gain your weight back. Here is one way to eat and not feel guilty.

Negative calorie foods are foods which require your body to use more energy to digest than the amount of calories in the food item itself. As a result, you will be able to enjoy both a nutritious food item, while burning calories at the same time.

Here is a list of some negative calorie foods[2]:

Negative Calorie Veggies

Asparagus – Beets – Broccoli – Cabbage (Green)
Carrots – Cauliflower – Celery – Chicory
Chili Peppers – Cucumbers – Dandelion –
Endive – Garden Cress – Garlic – Green Beans
Dark Green Leaf Lettuce – Onions – Radish –
Spinach – Turnip – Zucchini

Negative Calorie Fruits

Apples – Blueberries – Cantaloupe –
Cranberries – Grapefruit – Honeydew –
Lemons – Mangos – Oranges – Papaya –
Pineapple – Raspberries – Strawberries –
Tomato – Tangerines – Watermelon

2 (2004) *Body Building Pro: Negative Calorie Foods.* Retrieved from Body Building Pro Encyclopedia. Website: http://www.bodybuildingpro.com/negativecaloriefoods.html

– CHAPTER FIVE –

FIBER

from Andy

In July of 2001, I realized that Farm & Fleet did not have any jeans that would fit me if I got any bigger. I was wearing a size 44 and I weighed 263.5 pounds so I knew it was time to lose some weight. My wife suggested we try the Weight Watchers plan. I was allowed 28-35 points per day. So I decided to have a goal of 28 points because I really wanted to lose the weight. I also started walking one mile a day at the end of July.

I decided to stop drinking pop and Kool-Aid as I had been drinking about a gallon a day – which equals 1600 calories! Switching to water was not easy and it took a lot of willpower not to drink any Kool-Aid or pop. After sticking to the plan I lost 12 pounds in 5 days! Wow, this was working. By the following Friday I had lost 20 pounds and decided I needed a reward. So I ate Pizza until I could not move! But I knew I needed to get back on the plan and on Monday went into work and decided to see the health lady. She gave me some more tips and said I

Andy 's "before" photo in 2001

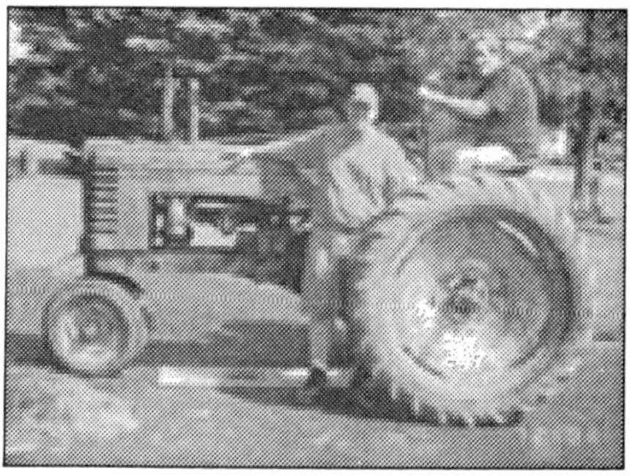

needed to pump my body full of fiber – at least 25 to 35 grams of fiber or more a day. I was eating maybe 10. She told me to get the fiber from fruits and vegetables, and Natural Ovens bread. Man this was great because I love bread – and now I could eat it and not gain weight.

I found out that I could eat a lot of food in a day. An example of a daily menu was a Natural Ovens' bagel for breakfast, three Gourmet Dinner rolls, apple or grapes, and Great Granola for lunch, a snack of granola at 3:00 and for supper I would have a small piece of meat, plain baked potato, corn or green beans and two pieces of Hunger Filler bread. I was getting 35-40 grams of fiber a day.

By working out an hour a day and walking three miles a day, rain or shine, I was losing a pound a day. Wow! I set my weight goal at 220 but my dad said, " Why not go for 200?" and I said, "Sure, why not". Once I was in the 230's I would treat myself to pizza or something "bad" for me. I was stuck on 227 for about six days, but I stayed with my high fiber, low fat plan and the next week I started losing again. Eating this way was becoming a habit.

I now fit into a size 34 pair of jeans and went from a 2XL shirt to a large. This was outstanding and everyone praised me and

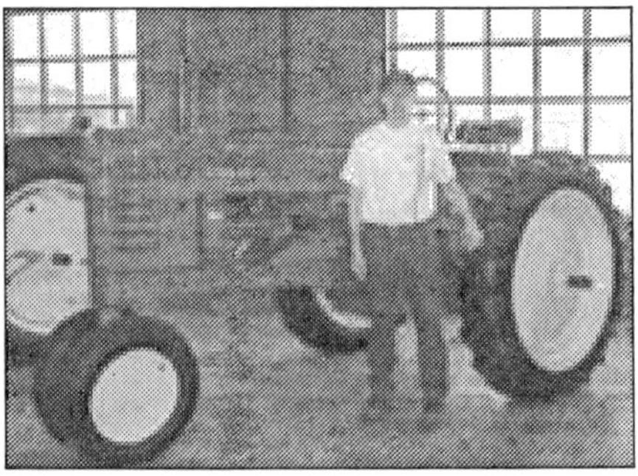

Andy's "after" photo in 2003

asked me how I did it. I thought maintaining could be hard, but it wasn't. I had grown to love these foods and I eat lots of Natural Ovens bread and other high fiber foods. I eat sweets in small portions rather than stuffing myself with them.

Over a year later I'm still eating about 35 grams of fiber a day and weigh between 170-175 pounds. This was a tremendous life change and I also think I might have been a prime candidate for diabetes. By eating lots of fiber, exercising, and drinking lots of water I will live longer and feel great. It's not a diet, it is a *lifestyle change.*

Andy South Beloit, IL

– CHAPTER SIX –

DIVIDE YOUR PLATE

from Susan

The first key to my weight loss has been a strategy entitled "Divide Your Plate." In this eating plan, you simply look at what you're eating and try to make half to two-thirds of what you eat fruits and vegetables. You make the remaining percentage low-fat protein and whole grains. Without realizing what I was doing, I cut out the empty carbs and lost my cravings for the crackers and pretzels that I had been eating every day. The main reason that this has worked is because it is **NOT** a diet. I don't count calories or carbs or points or anything. I just try to eat lots of fresh fruits and vegetables. They are colorful and tasty and crunchy and satisfying.

The second equally important key to my weight loss success has been an exercise program entitled, "8 Minutes in the Morning," by Jorge Cruise. Simply put, you do four sets of two exercises in the morning, six days a week. I did the "Week One" exercises for a few weeks in a row, and immediately started to notice results – both on the scale and in the way my clothes fit. I have been doing the exercises faithfully ever since. The exercises are simple and effective. I am stronger than I have ever been and especially enjoy being able to wave and not have that upper arm "arm jiggle."

My initial goal was to take off a stubborn 5 pounds that I just couldn't seem to lose with my regular walking. I ended up losing 20, and keeping it off. I went from a size 12 or 14 to a size 6 or 8. I have never felt more in shape or healthier. I find that now when I do snack on chips or a sweet, my body feels terrible. If I happen to skip a day of my exercises, I really miss it.

As I lost the weight and kept it off, I became more interested in healthy eating and how it "works." A friend told me about the Natural Ovens products, and I love the 100% Whole Grain Bread, especially when it is toasted. I also really like the Fruit and Lemon Great Granola Bars. I don't eat many bread products, but when I do, I try to make sure they are healthy ones.

I am currently 39 years old. By using the two strategies of "Divide Your Plate" and "8 Minutes in the Morning" I have no qualms about turning 40. I have never felt better!

Susan Edgerton, WI

– CHAPTER SEVEN –

QUALITY

from Andrew

I lost over 80 pounds with Natural Ovens breads! Deepest thanks to Natural Ovens Bakery for helping save my life. In August 2002, I reached a breaking point in my life. I weighed almost 300 pounds and was 47% body fat on a 5'10" frame at age 25. I was digging an early grave. So I entered a national fitness transformation contest with a strict food and exercise regimen. And I used Natural Ovens whole grain breads for all of my carb portions to help me get there. The key is quality in what you eat. And I cannot think of any other company today that's more concerned with its customers and the quality of its product, and not just the profit it makes. The real winners are the consumers, just look at the nutrition label and read the ingredients!

I am living proof that "low carb" diets, high protein diets, or any diet is bogus. The key word in diet is "Die". And who wants to feel like they

Andrew's "before" photo

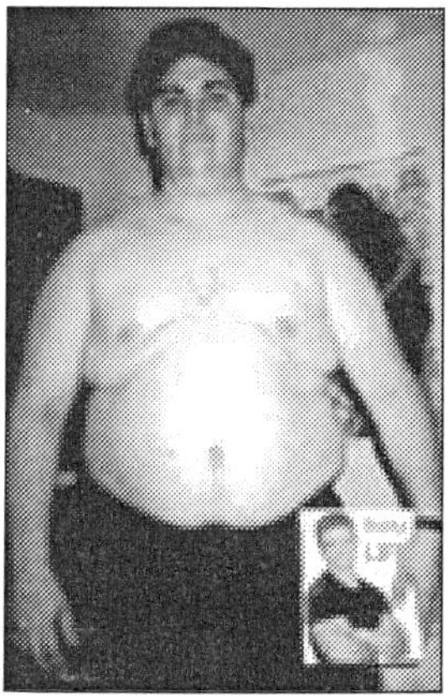

are dying? Today (July 2003), I weigh 212 pounds at 22% body fat, and have gained 10 pounds of muscle. I now plan on hitting 10% body fat before 2004. My newfound health has found my way to pursuing a black belt at Bally's Taekwondo Masters Academy in Brookfield, Wisconsin. I am a changed man, and I hope to shed light to others that your past does NOT have to equal your future!

Andrew Brookfield, WI

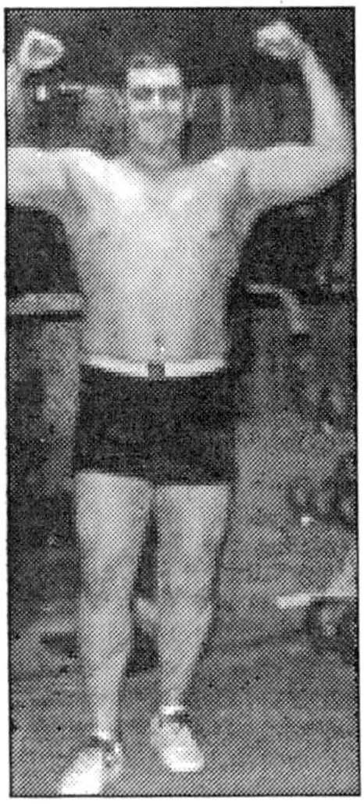

Andrew's "after" photo

– CHAPTER EIGHT –

CALORIES AND SERVING SIZES

from Jackie

When I was in my late 20's (now 37), I was unhappy and had low self-esteem about my body weight. I am 5'2" and was about 30 pounds overweight, which looks like 60 pounds overweight for my height. I was always the girl who couldn't eat whatever I wanted. Just smelling chocolate seemed to add poundage.

I finally decided to really regiment myself with diet and exercise. Since I enjoy quantity, I tried to find foods with as little calories as possible, so I could eat a lot of them. One thing I learned was to look at the product label for serving size after preparation. I was measuring uncooked rice and eating a lot of it and gaining weight, until I realized it was a measurement for already cooked rice. I was eating about four times the rice I was supposed to be eating. A typical day of eating for me would be:

Breakfast

1/3 cup uncooked oatmeal (Paul's Oats from Natural Ovens)

1/2 cup blueberries or 1 banana

Add real maple syrup, cinnamon, maple extract, powdered milk and water

Snack

The biggest Granny Smith apple I could find (they are the lowest calorie apple)

Some Fiber 1 cereal

Lunch

Natural Ovens bread for a turkey or tuna sandwich (no mayo, lots of mustard or salsa)

Snack

Air popped popcorn in a paper bag. (Seal with scotch tape and put in microwave)

Add a little spray butter and salt

Dinner

The biggest salad I could make using fresh veggies, cooked broccoli, and a protein. (Sometimes I used hard boiled eggs, a handful of nuts and raisins, turkey, chicken breast or tuna.)

Dessert

3 sugar free Fudgecicles*

This is about 1,000-1,200 calories for the day. I always keep hydrated with water. For exercising, I walk 5 miles at a fast pace every day. I like to do it for my mentality as well as for my body. I now have two small children who I need a lot of patience with. I pop in a favorite pre-recorded TV show in my VCR and walk on my treadmill, hopefully before anyone wakes up. Before children, I used to enjoy the city outdoors for my walks. I also do arm weights three days a week, and stomach exercises and stretching three days a week after my five mile walk. I only spend about an extra ten minutes a day.

I love what I eat and the way I feel after my workouts. Walking is pleasurable and not strenuous. It burns the most calories too.

I now have kept my weight down (except during pregnancies) and am always working at maintaining my weight. It's never easy, but I wouldn't want to go back to the way I used to look ever again. You just have to remember that this is a change in your foods for *life*, not just a temporary diet change.

Jackie Glen Ellyn, IL

– CHAPTER NINE –

A FEW HELPFUL HINTS

from Julie

As a registered nurse and someone who is committed to making healthy choices, I would like to share a few of my own suggestions that have helped me in my weight loss.

1. Avoid skipping meals as skipping can cause cravings for processed and high glycemic index foods.

2. Eat ample fresh fruits, vegetables, whole grains, and high fiber and low fat protein foods to satisfy yourself.

3. Trade in the large dinner plate for a smaller version and limit second helpings.

4. Have fresh fruits and vegetables washed and within easy reach for snacking urges.

5. Never shop on an "empty" stomach as this impairs decision-making and helps sugary snacks find their way into your cart.

6. Drink a glass of water before each meal for hydration and to promote fullness.

7. Exercise for at least 30 minutes daily, and this will soon become a habit. Once endurance improves, try to exercise for more than 30 minutes.

8. Avoid being critical of yourself. It is very easy to slip and make an unhealthy choice from time to time. Just remember that you can start your day over at any time.

Shedding extra pounds and keeping them off takes effort and discipline. These tips have helped me and they may help you see results as well.

Julie Shorewood, WI

– CHAPTER TEN –

THE LEAN PLATE CLUB: SUPERSIZE THAT SALAD[3]

Imagine adding a super-sized course to your meal that actually trims calories from the bottom line. You probably think it's too good to be true. Wrong again.

Findings presented by Pennsylvania State University researchers at the annual meeting of the North American Association for the Study of Obesity found that starting lunch with a healthy salad reduced the total calories people consumed in the meal. The seven-week study of 42 people found that participants who ate three cups of low-calorie salad as a first course wound up eating fewer calories at the meal than those who skipped the salad.

"The findings are surprising because usually adding variety to a meal by adding an extra course tends to make people eat more," said Barbara Rolls, professor of nutrition at Penn State and lead author of the study. Here's how to apply these results to daily life:

Keep it low-fat. The study looked at six salads varying in size, calories and fat. The lowest-fat salads -- those with 14 percent of calories from fat -- worked best at reducing overall food consumption. Have your dressing on the side, dip your fork in the dressing, and then take your bite of salad – surprisingly satisfying.

Size matters. In the study, larger salads were better than smaller ones at shaving calories from the meal. Eating three cups of low-fat salads resulted in a 12 percent overall reduction in lunch calories compared with 7 percent fewer calories for those who ate 1-1/2 cups of salad. Best (and most surprising) news: Participants felt equally full on three cups of salad, whether it contained 100 or 400 calories.

Watch the tipping point. The study found that a salad of about 100 calories had the most effect at reducing overall calories for the meal. As calories crept to 200, with moderate fat, there was either no change in total meal calorie consumption or a slight increase in calories. High-fat salads of 200 calories or more actually resulted in higher total calories at lunch, up to 145 more. That's another reason, Rolls says, to load up on the low-cal veggies -- and not the cheese and (high-fat) dressing. Vinaigrettes are lower in calories and higher in flavor than most other salad dressings.

Pile on the greens. They're filled with flavor, water, fiber and plenty of phytonutrients, minerals and vitamins and have about five calories per cup. Plus, three cups of greens provide three of the nine servings per day of fruit and vegetables recommended by the Institute for Cancer Research. In the study, salads were made of Romaine lettuce, carrots, tomatoes, celery and cucumbers (as well as small amounts dressing). But any combination of greens and other water-filled vegetables will likely do. "The bigger the vegetable volume, the bigger the impact of this first course," Rolls says.

Savor the flavor. Participants in the study got 20 minutes to eat their first-course salads -- more than many people take to eat their entire lunch at their desks. Research suggests that eating slowly gives your stomach time to send satiety signals to the brain.

Ask for the dressing on the side. That puts portion control in your court, not the restaurants. Study participants got one to three tablespoons of dressing on their salads -- far less than most restaurants slather on -- yet they still reported feeling full afterward. "The fullness wasn't affected by the calories, only by the portion," Rolls says.

Add real whole grain toasted croutons. Can't buy them? Make them by toasting whole grain bread that has at least 3 grams of fiber per slice. Whole grains add long term satiety to any salad to keep you from getting hungry for hours.

What's a Serving?

What counts towards 9-A-Day? All varieties of fruits and vegetables - fresh, frozen, dried and 100 percent juice. A serving size is smaller than many people think. The Institute for Cancer Research co-sponsor of the 9-A-Day for Better Health program, defines a serving as:

- One medium-sized fruit (ex. apple, orange, banana, pear)
- 1/2 cup of raw, cooked, or frozen fruits or vegetables
- 3/4 cup (6 oz.) of 100 percent fruit or vegetable juice
- 1/2 cup cut-up fresh fruit

- 1/2 cup cooked or canned legumes (beans and peas)
- 1 cup of raw, leafy vegetables (ex. Romaine lettuce, spinach)
- 1/4 cup dried fruit (ex. raisins, apricots, mango)

Be creative when eating your nine servings of fruits and vegetables every day.

– CHAPTER ELEVEN –

SUGARBUSTERS

from Nancy

It has been five or six years now since both my husband and I have lost 40-50 pounds each. We are now in our early 60's and I needed to do this for health reasons.

While shopping, a *Sugarbusters* book almost fell off the shelf and into my cart. I took that as a sign – and I did a modest version of it. The book made a lot of sense to me.

We eliminated sugary foods with more than 3 grams of sugar. That is no longer the toughest thing to do with all the products on the market today. It is very eye opening to see how much sugar is added to things you normally wouldn't suspect.

We have limited carbs to whole grains with as little processing as possible. Instead of potatoes we now eat brown rice, lentils, barley and lots of beans. And usually it is about 1/4 cup a serving. Because they have more flavors and are chewier, it is easy to abide by the 1/4 cup measure. We have also refused to buy anything with hydrogenated fats.

We remember to eat a mid morning snack of fresh fruit or raw nuts and again in mid afternoon – this eliminates ravenous appetites at lunch and dinner.

We never eat after 8 pm at night when calories have fewer chances of being burned. Bread is limited to Natural Ovens "Hunger Filler" or an occasional slice of "Happiness" bread. And of course, a box of Paul's Oatmeal is always in reach.

We walk a mile or more on most days and participate in a senior aerobics class twice a week for 3/4's of the year. The pounds have stayed off and life is good. Thanks to Natural Ovens Bakery for providing a healthy "Staff of Life." It has been of great help!

Nancy Green Bay, WI

– CHAPTER TWELVE –

TRIGGER POINT

from Jessica

I have successfully stayed the same weight for the past three years after losing over 100 pounds. My "trigger point" was many different things that just started to add up. My daughter wanted to go on bike rides; I couldn't walk the neighborhood with my neighbor without feeling like I was going to pass out, stairs were very difficult for me, and I was tired all of the time. I realized that I was too young to be feeling so old and I didn't like who I was. I had tried many different diets all of my life with some success, but eventually just gained the weight back. I started in the Weight Watcher program, which is where I learned of Natural Ovens Bakery products and stayed with WW for approximately nine months. Financially it was difficult for me to stay in the program and I promised myself that if I went back to bad eating habits I would have to go back into the program. After that, I created my own way of eating.

I try to eat very well balanced meals, completely eliminating all meats except fish from my diet and I really try to stay away from most trans-fat products or refined sugars and flours. I also have eliminated all fast food restaurants from my diet. My family eats what I eat and I can also see a healthier change in them. We eat a lot of beans, brown rice, and whole grain products. Fruits and vegetables are at almost every meal. I also drink approximately 120 ounces of water every day; it is amazing how different I feel if I don't drink enough water during the day. As I stated earlier, I am also a huge believer in the Natural Ovens' products. I buy at least 3 to 4 products a week and can't remember the last time a bought a "regular" loaf of bread. Bagels, breads, cookies, and their great granola bars make up most of what I buy. Often times I have to travel to three different stores in my area to find the products I want for the week, which has become a family joke, but it is that important to me.

With all the diet fads out there right now, I really believe that most everything is okay if it is done in moderation. I don't eliminate carbs or other things, but I do choose good foods. Something that really helps me during the day, especially my work day, is having snacks available so that I am not tempted by other things. I usually have fruit, yogurt, Natural Ovens' cookies or granola bars with me.

I also exercise regularly, usually four to five times a week. *When I first started I could barely do 10 minutes of an easy exercise video, now I walk, run, work on machines at our fitness club, and do aerobic tapes.* It is a part of my everyday routine and I miss it if I don't try to fit it in somewhere.

I actually dislike some of the foods I used to eat, because I am more aware of what certain ingredients do to my body. I read every label. However there are certain things I won't give up (favorite – ice cream), but instead of eating a whole container myself, we go out for a cone. (Editors note: Check the Natural Food Section and try the soy or rice dream ice creams as they do not contain animal hormones.)

Finally, feeling good about myself is my best motivator. I can keep up with my daughter and even beat her in a race up a hill sometimes! *And after going down eight clothing sizes, I also can shop at almost any clothing store which is a big treat for me.* Most people who have not seen me for some time hardly recognize me and almost all want to know my secret. Truth is, there is no secret. Eating well balanced meals of good-for-you food, drinking plenty of water and getting exercise is all you need to know. I think it would be helpful to people to be more aware of what they eat and what it does to their overall health.

Jessica Minnesota

– CHAPTER THIRTEEN –

SIZE 4 EQUALS SIZE 0[4]

On January 20, 2004 the New York Times published an article by one of our favorite nutrition writers, Jane E. Brody. Her outstanding article was titled: *The Widening of America, or How Size 4 Became a Size 0.*

She stated, "Last fall, I was thrilled to find a pair of size 0 cotton stretch slacks that fit perfectly. Now, I have never been a 0, not since puberty anyway. I am, at best, a size 4, which is two sizes smaller than what I wore at the same weight in the 1970's." What has happened? Size inflation, that's what.

Women — and men — who have packed on the pounds want to be able to wear the same sizes they wore in their trimmer days years ago. So the fashion industry accommodated, with today's size 4 fitting like former size 8, 8 like 12, 12 like 16 and so forth.

Men's slacks once labeled "regular" are now "slim cut," and for those who cannot squeeze into those, there are easy fit, loose fit and baggy fit. Greg Critser, in his illuminating book *Fat Land: How Americans Became the Fattest People in the World* (Mariner Books paperback, $13), points out, "The new cuts were in reality simply bigger sizes, without the bigger numbers."

New Yorkers complain that the subway cars, many of them made in Japan, can seat one-third fewer people than they were meant to.

4 Brody, J. (2004, January 20). The Widening of America, or How Size 4 Became a Size 0. *New York Times*

Why? Because the typical seated American covers a lot more bench than a Japanese commuter. In response to a complaint from an oversize customer, the president of the Olive Garden restaurant chain ordered bigger chairs, lest the biggest eaters decide to dine elsewhere.

Americans live in a land of abundance where super sizing can be a necessity if you want to stay in business, be it movie theater popcorn, fast food, soft drinks or automobiles. A McDonald's meal that once had 540 calories now packs in 1,550. The items are the same, but the portions have tripled. And studies have shown that even if people are satisfied with less, they will eat more if portions are larger.

Even dieters, it seems, want to eat as much as they can without having to pay a caloric price for their indulgence. How else can anyone explain the enormous popularity of Atkins-like diets that promise weight loss without deprivation as long as the dieter sticks to a low-carbohydrate regimen — as many cheeseburgers as wanted, but without buns or ketchup; bacon and sausage with the cheese omelet but no toast; and gobs of fatty dressing on the salad but no croutons.

People do lose weight on these diets. How? Because they eat less than they did before (as one lapsed Atkins dieter remarked, "What's a burger without a bun?"). Because they cannot indulge in 400-calorie bagels, 600-calorie muffins, Krispy Kreme doughnuts, Haagen-Dazs ice cream, pies, cakes, cookies or even rice, white pasta, white bread or potatoes. Nor can they grab a candy bar or down a sugary soda when the snack bug bites.

A healthy body does not waste calories. If you eat them, your body counts them, and if you eat more calories than you use, you gain weight, not lose it, no matter what the contents of the diet.

– CHAPTER FOURTEEN –

CHILDREN AT RISK

With each consecutive survey, the number of overweight Americans increases. More than 60 percent of adults and 20 percent of children are now overweight or obese. When will it end? Not soon, if dietary habits and sedentary trends continue.

In a national study of 6,212 children and adolescents published in the current issue of the journal Pediatrics, researchers at the Agriculture Department and the Harvard Medical School found that on a typical day 30.3 percent of the people surveyed reported eating fast food. The people who ate fast food that day consumed 187 more calories, 9 more grams of fat, 26 more grams of added sugars, 228 more grams of sugar-sweetened drinks and less fiber, fruits and non-starchy vegetables than youngsters who did not eat fast food that day.

Not only did the fast-food eaters consume more calories, but they also ate fewer health-sustaining nutrients.

As Mr. Critser points out, schools from kindergarten through college are complicit in the galloping epidemic of obesity. Overburdened and underfinanced school systems throughout the country have invited fast-food purveyors and soft-drink vending machines to their premises, often with monetary or equipment kickbacks from the producers.

The push to raise academic scores has squeezed out many physical education programs and athletic activities, not to mention art and music. After school outdoor activities have yielded to computers, video games and television, the modern-day baby sitters. A result is increasing numbers of youngsters who are eating more and moving less — and putting on fat cells that will be with them for life.

I am often asked why the food industry produces so many products that can undermine health. The answer is simple. Because people buy them. Any food item that does not sell soon disappears from the marketplace. The industry supplies what consumers demand. If more people eating fast food choose salads over fries, the salad choices in those establishments will increase. (Editor's note: Of course, making these foods so *addictive* has played a huge role in having so many products on the market.)

If parents unite and demand a change in school lunch offerings or if more children take lunch from home, childhood nutrition will improve. Parents must remind school authorities that a sound mind has to reside in a sound body; children's physical development should not be sacrificed to academic scores.

(Editor's note: Are you interested in improving the foods in your schools? Call 1-800-772-0730 and order a copy of the *Roadmap for Healthy Foods in Schools* ($25 including shipping and handling) The "Roadmap" contains 75 pages of instruction with recipes, sample menus, and a 14-minute dynamite DVD depicting 6 years experience with the Appleton, Wisconsin Central Alternative School. The students improved so much in behavior and academic ability that the program was adapted in the entire school district and 15,000 students now have healthier foods!)

– CHAPTER FIFTEEN –

ANSWERS

Start putting pressure on the big food companies and fast food chains. Write to corporate headquarters about nutrition concerns and, if possible, offer suggestions for alternative products and urge a reduction in portion sizes. You might also voice your support for a tax on snack items and a ban on television advertising on children's programs for nutritionally questionable foods, for example, those that exceed a certain fat or sugar ratio to healthful nutrients.

The recent suits by obese youngsters against McDonald's may sound laughable, because no one forced the youngsters to eat that fattening fare. But the negative publicity that the suits attract to the company's high-calorie offerings may help others stop eating them before they, too, balloon into obesity. Look what citizens' suits against tobacco companies have wrought.

An end result may be legislation that requires food companies to advertise healthy eating plans. Currently, Mr. Critser points out, "The soft drink industry alone spends upward of $600 million annually to promote its trash, compared with the National Cancer Institute's paltry $1 million budget for promoting fruit and vegetable consumption."

– CHAPTER SIXTEEN –

SWEET TOOTH

from Nancy

I lost 35 pounds and have kept it off for 1 year. I am 53 years old, was always slender until my 40's when I started slowly putting on the pounds, and then had a rapid (over maybe a year) weight gain totalling 35-40 pounds of excess weight. I was put on Elavil for postoperative pain, and this medication 'assisted' an already terrific sweet-tooth. I've always been an out of control sweet eater. I eventually went from 127 to 165 pounds and felt and looked terrible. (I take full responsibility for eating Fanny May candy every day.)

I lost my job in June 2003, and decided to take the opportunity to go on Seattle Sutton's Healthy Eating (SSHE) diet – the 1200 calorie/day version. It would have been tough doing this while working – I'm a project engineer, was very busy and grabbed food when I had time. I lost 35 pounds in exactly 3 months. Also, my personal motivator was that in October, 2003, I traveled to Delaware with my husband to meet my birth-father for the first time, and didn't want him to meet me looking so different than I always had my whole life.

I was 'starved' most of the time I was on the SSHE diet. I never cheated except that I ate dinner at my son's wedding (with cake). I attended his bridal shower and didn't eat (except for a small piece of cake – you can tell my weakness). My husband said he was impressed with my will power. I think my body was craving the sweets I'd lived on for years.

I now weigh myself almost every day so I don't gain too much weight (I fluctuate 2-3 pounds). I've eaten Natural Ovens bread on sandwiches and toast (Happiness) for maybe 10 years, but now it's a major component of my healthy diet. It's high in fiber (therefore filling), great tasting, has no trans fats, has Omega-3, etc. I do not exercise on an organized basis, but we have a dog I walk 3-4 times/day for maybe a total of an hour.

I still love sweets (mostly dark chocolate candy), but can no longer stand all the trans fats I used to eat in pastries, pie crusts, crackers, etc. I am a fanatic about checking labels in the grocery store, and inform my husband about what I find. Sometimes I think just reading so much about partially hydrogenated trans fats has turned me off to them.

The two most important things that have kept my weight off (other than eating healthier) is that I now drink a lot more water than I used to, and we eat out in restaurants much less frequently. We're empty nesters and for a number of years ate most meals out. *The portions are always too big,* and they generally use more sodium, trans fats, etc. than I do at home. (Editor's note: A great solution to eating out is for each to have a mixed salad and split one main course. Your waiter will be happy to supply you with extra small plates as this is quite common now.)

I feel so much better at this lower weight than I did. Although I wasn't obese, even climbing stairs was harder than when I am slimmer.

Nancy Florida

– CHAPTER SEVENTEEN –

FIFTEEN POUNDS

from Rebecca

I have never been very heavy until about 3 or 4 years ago when I weighed about 15 pounds more than I do now. I was not active, rarely exercised, and ate essentially whatever I wanted to. I think if it were not for youth and good genes I would have been extremely overweight. For whatever reason, I realized that my lifestyle was not healthy, and that I needed to change.

I began running just 1-1/2 miles a few times a week, cutting out the potato chips and candy bars, and monitoring my portion sizes. I tried vegetables that I thought I would never like, and found I loved them! The weight loss was gradual, and I think that has played a big role in my being able to keep the weight off easily.

I think that anyone who truly wants to lose weight should never be too drastic too fast. Slowly cutting out the bad foods and replacing them with good things is important. And I do not believe anyone can lose weight and keep it off without some kind of exercise, even if it only means walking to the cleaners versus driving. That is better than not exercising at all.

Foods that used to comfort me now revolt me. I have not eaten a potato chip or a candy bar in 3 years. I do get sweet cravings and I try to satisfy them with a low fat oatmeal raisin cookie or fruit. I love bread so I eat Natural Ovens Right Wheat or Hunger Filler. Mornings are not mornings without cereal so I eat Paul's Oats from Natural Ovens or high fiber Kashi.

There are certain things that I just simply have to say no to, and be disciplined not to eat them. There are days when the last thing I want to do is run or go to kickboxing. But for the most part I joyfully embrace this healthy lifestyle. That is the key to losing weight and keeping it off. Find whatever works for you, whatever you can be happy with and be excited about, and stick with it. Get your husband, friend, sister, or even your pet involved if that is what it takes, *but make exercise a part of your life.*

Rebecca Libertyville, IL

– CHAPTER EIGHTEEN –

FAST FOOD NATION

We thought you may enjoy this excerpt from *Fast Food Nation.*

> Life is more hectic than ever -- between school, sports, clubs and friends, who has time to think about what to eat? Time for plan B: fast food. "Fast food is easy," said Sarah Hudson, a 14-year-old from Portland, Maine. "It's quick and it tastes good." She figures she eats fast food about twice a week. "As long as it tastes good and it fills you up then that's all I care about," said her friend Ryan Bell, 13. "We buy it because it tastes good. If they made healthy food I doubt we would buy it."

(Editor's Note: Read *Beating the Food Giants* by Paul Stitt to learn about the wide use of appetite stimulants that make you "think" the fast foods taste good.)

The average American now consumes about three hamburgers and four orders of French fries every week. That's 90 grams of fat and 2,520 calories. The average person needs about 2,000 calories for a whole day. Most Americans know that fast food isn't exactly good for them, but can't quite seem to break the habit. In fact, consumption of high-fat fast food is increasing, in part because fast food restaurants are an inescapable part of American life.

According to *Fast Food Nation*, a great book by Eric Schlosser, 96 percent of American schoolchildren can identify Ronald McDonald. The only fictional character with a higher degree of recognition is Santa Claus. Schlosser says it's nearly impossible to overstate the impact of the fast food industry on the nation's culture, economy and diet. "McDonald's Golden Arches," he writes, "are now more widely recognized than the Christian cross." Considering America's love of the French fry, it's no surprise that kids are getting bigger. The percentage of children and teenagers who are overweight has tripled in the past 30 years, according to the Center for Disease Control. One-third of overweight students are so heavy they will probably have serious health problems later in life.

Of course it's not just young people who are getting heavier -- it's all Americans. U.S. Surgeon General Dr. David Satcher is so concerned about childhood obesity that he has declared it an "epidemic." "We see a nation of young people seriously at risk of starting out obese and dooming themselves to the difficult task of overcoming a tough illness," he said. He's not talking about kids who are chubby or a little plump. These are kids who are more than 20 percent above their ideal weight -- kids whose weight makes it hard for them to move around, get up stairs and even breathe.

Doctors are finding that more and more severely overweight children have medical problems such as a fatty liver, a precursor to liver disease, high blood pressure, and an increasing likelihood of Type 2 diabetes. In addition, obese children are becoming prime candidates for heart attacks and strokes even while in their teens. Researchers say it's important to realize that obesity is a health problem -- not a judgment about how people's bodies should look. Everyone has their own idea about how they like to look, but nobody wants to have a heart attack.

How can you tell if you are overweight, obese, or just about right? How do you feel? Ideal weight is usually given in a range of at least 15 pounds. If you have a small frame, you should probably be toward the bottom of the range. And, logically, the opposite for bigger people. If you are more than a few pounds above your ideal weight, you are overweight. But if you are more than 20 percent above your ideal weight, you are obese. That means your weight could start to destroy your health.

Weight is strongly influenced by genes -- you are more likely to be heavy if your parents are heavy, especially if you also inherited their eating habits. But, there is something you can do. Doctors say the most important way for kids and adults to lose weight is to change their eating habits. That means finding an alternative to all-night pizza delivery, convenience stores, and fast food restaurants.

Sometimes it's even hard to find nutritious foods in school, where many cafeterias have been replaced with mall-style food courts. Many schools across the country have also signed contracts with soft drink companies like Coke and Pepsi. The schools agree to install soda machines and the school must guarantee a set number of sales in order for the schools to get their "money". Schools often use the money from these contracts for teacher salaries and special programs but such contracts often require schools to sell as many as 50 sodas per student per school year.

Recent studies by the US Agriculture Department now link obesity to soft drink consumption for the first time. The studies show that students drink soda instead of eating healthy meals, and then eat more food later because they are not filled up. So students are drinking more sugar and syrup and eating more food than they would if they just ate a regular lunch.

As doctors, teachers, parents and kids try to work on developing healthy eating and exercise habits, there's also the danger that some kids will go too far. Many kids of normal weight seem to think they're fat -- and can develop eating disorders that are just as dangerous to their health as diabetes and stroke.

– CHAPTER NINETEEN –

FOUR KEY FACTORS

from Rachel

I am one of the success stories as far as weight loss goes. My doctor said he wants to use me as an example to other patients he has. I lost a total of 70 pounds so far, and would actually like to lose another 5. I am pregnant right now, so that's on hold for the time being (but let me tell you, my pregnancy has been very trouble free and I didn't have to adjust a thing as far as how I eat.)

I started this whole journey to better health in 1996. And I did it not by any fad diet, pills, or anything out of the ordinary. I simply ate healthier and less food, and increased how much I exercised.

There are actually 4 main things that I feel helped me to change my lifestyle.

1) Prayer – as a believer in Jesus Christ, I realized that I had been trying my whole life to lose weight to no avail, but I needed the power of God to help me stay disciplined in my eating habits,

2) Accountability – I found that (sort of by accident) being in a group with other women who were trying to eat healthier, and who were weighing in once a week, really gave me the support and encouragement I needed to start losing weight,

3) Attitude change – I had to learn what my destructive eating habits were and eliminate them, and to realize that I can't just eat what-

ever or whenever I want. Just like any other problem people face, like anger for example, it needs to be controlled,

4) Written record/Discipline – for me I needed to write down everything I ate in a day to keep track so I didn't try to fool myself. As a matter of fact, 8 years later, I'm still writing down everything I eat in a day.

I actually plan out a week in advance so I know exactly what I want to eat when. This helps me at the grocery store too because I make a list and stick to it. Then there's no other "junk food in the house to throw me off. Then, I needed to follow the plan. Sure, holidays, or summer picnics, or church potlucks come up. And I allowed myself an occasional splurge (like on my birthday I had chocolates and lobster dinner complete with a piece of birthday cake at the end). But, I try to plan in those special events too, and if I fail, I don't worry about it, I just get back to the plan the next meal, or the next day. This is a plan for life and things are going to come up. I think that attitude has also helped me stay on track. The weight has come off probably more slowly, but I understand that is good to helping to keep the weight off.

Rachel's "before" photo

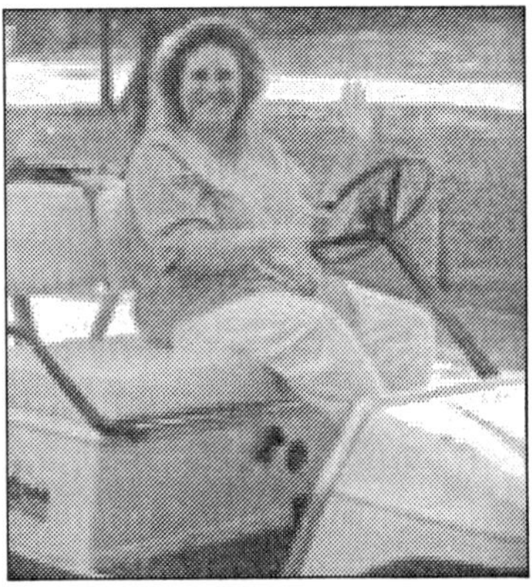

I started this because I always wanted to be thinner, but what kicked me into gear was I wanted to be healthier. I saw my relatives with high blood pressure and adult onset diabetes struggling to change their eating habits, and figured I needed to change my habits young if I was going to be successful. So, I followed a plan that is loosely based on a suggested "exchange" based eating plan by the American Diabetes Association.

I had to learn a little bit about calories and how proteins and carbohydrates interact, and what constitutes an "exchange." But, basically, in a day I try to eat 3 servings of fruit, at least 2 servings of vegetables, 4 or less servings of protein, 4 (I started with 6 but to keep losing I now go with 4) servings of starchy complex carbohydrates, 3 or less servings of fat, and at least 8 cups of water (I actually drink about a gallon of water everyday). And I do it in 6 smaller servings (3 meals and 3 snacks) about 2-1/2-3 hours apart each day.

I found this eating plan took some change of attitude and adjustment. I had to learn to like foods that were good for me – like carrots (most vegetables). And to eat foods that were bad for me less often and in smaller quantities –

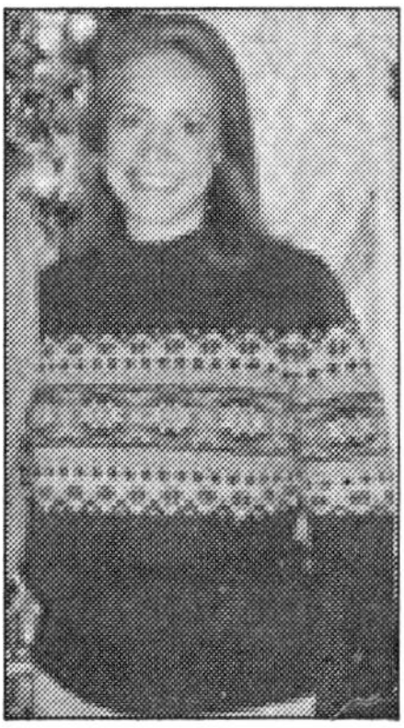

Rachel's "after" photo

like pizza. But other than fast food (I can't believe the fat and calories in that stuff – it just wasn't worth it to me) I didn't eliminate anything from my diet. I merely cut back. Pizza is a good example.

My husband and I used to order 2 medium pizzas at a place and each eat one. Now, if we have pizza, I try to stick to 2 pieces. I also changed the types of food I was eating. For example, instead of squishy white bread that offers little to no nutritional value, I began eating Natural Ovens' bread. Instead of boxed processed foods, I began to make my own casseroles or whatever using healthier ingredients. I do try to stay away from the packaged weight loss products too. Because again, this is a life plan for better health and some of those products that promise all kinds of weight loss, low-fat or whatever benefits, actually have a lot of chemicals that our bodies don't need either. Food that grows out of the ground seemed the better and healthier way to go.

I did find my tastes changed. I have a new appreciation for a lot of fruits. Sometimes fruit satisfies a sweet craving I might have – and that's saying a lot for me, the candy and cookie lover. Even foods I didn't like before (mostly vegetables) I found I acquired a taste for if I just gave them a chance.

Of course the intake of calories would not be complete without the expending of the calories. I changed my exercise habits too. I had been exercising some for many years. But I increased or changed the amount and intensity. I began walking. Then I thought I would like to try jogging. It was slow at first. I had to jog a block and then walk a block and jog a block, etc.

I got to the point where I would be able to jog half the distance and then the whole distance. I found I loved jogging.

The height, so far for me was when I finished an organized 15K run (almost 10 miles) at a personal best time. I'm considering half marathons or marathons, but I don't know if I want to commit the time (especially with a new family about to arrive). And, I began to bike too. Not extensively long distances. But it just gives me an extra boost in my exercise program. I try to bike places that I was going anyway that way it only takes a little extra time instead of planning a whole bike trip I wasn't planning in the first place.

Biking or walking are healthy activities the whole family can do together. So I know exercise is different for everybody, but I know everybody can find something that will increase their activity level that they are able to do and enjoy doing – you just have to get out and try things – walking, swimming, jogging, biking, sports, aerobic classes or tapes, etc. I also lift weights about every other day. I'm not a body builder, but just try to keep toned, strong and in shape.

Finally motivation is a big key. I tend to be a disciplined person by nature. So sometimes, just having a plan keeps me on track. But, my biggest weakness in life is fast food. So, eating right tends to be the hardest thing for me to stay disciplined in. Some of the day to day practical things I've found that help to motivate me are:

1) Success – when I would see the scale go down a pound, I was elated and motivated to do it again. I weigh myself once a week and I write it down. I know that many factors influence weight gain or loss from week to week. So, I look

for a pattern over time, overall and don't live or die by the scale. But, it is a gauge that helps me see where I am.

2) Encouragement from others – mostly my husband. He has been a great source of encouragement and now has lost 45 pounds himself just over the last year. The biggest part of his success in the beginning was just cutting out sugared soda. I urge everyone to get at least one cheerleader to help them stay encouraged – no discipline seems pleasant when you're going through it, but it produces a great result, and having someone there to remind you of what you've accomplished is helpful.

3) Having to buy new clothes. There was nothing more exciting to me than watching the clothes sizes I was getting into get smaller and smaller. And, I recommend that to the best your budget allows, buy new smaller clothes that you really like and get rid of the old bigger ones. It helps remind you to stay that size because you don't want to have to buy bigger clothes again.

4) Setting goals. Having healthy goals to shoot for like a time on an organized run, or a distance you'd like to walk, or that you won't go off your eating plan for three days, or that you're going to change one processed food to one healthy food this week, or whatever. These are all steps in the right direction. And not getting destroyed by failed goals, but just getting right back into it.

Remember, this is a health plan for life, not a fad diet, not a temporary thing. So, any steps toward better health are good steps, but don't be afraid to shoot for high goals either. You might actually reach them.

Rachel Sheboygan, WI

– CHAPTER TWENTY –

NEW HOLE

from Dave

I have lost about 8 to 10 pounds which isn't easy since I was at 159 to start. I think I started around August of last year, so it isn't a long term thing, as of yet. I remember Paul Stitt, then President of Natural Ovens, talking about nutrition, etc. at a PaceSetters running club meeting a long time ago in Kimberly. What he was saying at that time, I was laughing about. Being thick headed, I went my own way for many years. Then I started walking intensely as I was laid off for two weeks. It was like a light bulb went off in my brain. I remembered the things he said, and went to Natural Ovens website www.naturalovens.com for advice.

Remembering what Paul said I changed my diet. I gave up a life time of drinking milk, soda, and caffeine coffee. I switched to water and decaf. I stopped eating deep fat fried foods and I now go to Subway if I am on the road. I started drinking water at meals and stopped eating white bread, and started eating breakfast of high fiber cereal. I eat a lot of dark green leafy lettuce salads almost every day, if I can. I started walking every day and mostly what helped was watching what I ate and trying to adjust my lifestyle.

I just wanted to say thanks for all the advice. I never thought much of the Adkins diet, because I feel a need for fiber and proper elemination. I feel better and hope I look better too. It was kind of mental to deal with giving up certain foods. It was also hard to not think of all the good times at certain restaurants which I enjoyed. But the longer you stick with it, the easier it is. My pants are baggier and I have had to put a new hole in my belt. I have tried to stay on track and not fall off, but sometimes I stumble and eat the wrong things. But I just focus and eat better the next day.

Dave Appleton, WI

– CHAPTER TWENTY ONE –

VITAMIN/MINERAL DEFICIENCY

from Alexandra

In April of 2002 at the ripe old age of just 31 I was diagnosed with rosacea. No doctor seemed able to tell me what causes it. I did a lot of research and found that it stems from the blood vessels being too close to the surface of the skin due to an inflammatory response (to what no one knows) and that the blood vessels had lost elasticity. Further research and I learned that loss of elasticity of blood vessels was most likely due to certain vitamin and mineral deficiencies that cause the body to not be able to produce enough collagen. Since I had always thought I was eating healthy and usually took a multivitamin I couldn't understand how I could be vitamin/mineral deficient. From here I learned about the concept of whole foods and that I wasn't really eating healthy before.

I learned what it meant to, for example, strip the bran and germ from wheat, make pasta out of it only putting back five of the nutrients, and when your body goes to try to use the energy from that pasta it finds it doesn't have all the micronutrients to utilize that energy and it leeches those from elsewhere in your body, leading to all sorts of perhaps small to nearly unnoticeable signs of minor malnutrition like skin problems, or bad hair and nails, or weight gain or inability to lose weight.

I learned all about sugar and its devastating effects on all aspects of health from the insulin yo yo to the immune system, and more. I bought the book *The Healing Power of Whole Foods* which in reality glossed quickly over the science behind whole foods but it was a great resource for recipes and had a fantastic index of what foods and ingredients were or weren't whole foods. From here I also began learning about stress and all the effects being in a constant "fight or flight" state has on health.

With all this new information on nutrition, I became a label reader. Grocery shopping often took an hour and a half or more as I read the labels on everything I picked, often having to put it all right back. It was hard to find, for example, prepared pasta sauces that did not have added sugars or MSG (we also went MSG free, another complication for grocery shopping as there are so many other names it can go by).

It took some time, but we finally got into a groove with what foods and what brands to buy and at which grocery stores often driving an hour into the city to get some foods that were not available at our local grocery store's natural food section. We cut out as much sugar as we could, we switched to 100% whole wheat pasta, brown rice, we never peel potatoes anymore, and we were already eating Natural Ovens' whole grain Great Granola and breads.

Buying prepared cereals were a toughie, my step-sons didn't take well to our new way of life and so we bought the healthiest alternatives we could for them keeping the sugar per serving at 6g or less, cereals like those from Enviorkids have been going over well with them like Cheetah Chomps and Peanut Butter Bumpers. We don't drink pop any more though we know the kids get it when they are not home. Instead we keep Knudsen's fruit juice Spritzers around as a healthier alternative though still not a whole food. We also switched to goat's milk for all the obvious reason that I won't go into here. We had to curtail our eating out as there was really no eating healthy when eating out. Cooking from scratch became the norm as it was the only way to ensure we were getting whole foods and no MSG or sugar. I began drinking iced tea especially when we did go out to eat. I also started taking a three-a-day type whole food multi-vitamin and tried to work on de-stressing.

While switching to a whole foods lifestyle first came about in an effort to battle rosacea it turned into a quest for better health in general, and weight loss has ended up just being a bonus to this new eating style. While it has been slow, I have lost about 20 pounds or so and it has stayed off. My rosacea is under control with my skin being almost like it was before 2002 and my husband and I feel so much healthier in general.

Alexandra Glencoe, MN

CHAPTER TWENTY TWO

NEW STUDY SUGGESTS CONSUMERS WOULD LIKE TO EAT HEALTHIER FOOD[5]

Consumers are demanding healthier foods, according to a new study released by the Food Marketing Institute and *Prevention* magazine. The release of the new report, "Shopping for Health 2004," comes as the U.S. Department of Agriculture prepares to unveil its new Dietary Guidelines for Americans in early 2005. Those guidelines likely will shake up food intake recommendations in an effort to improve the nation's health. According to the study, consumers have begun paying more attention to nutrition labels, purchasing more organic foods for health benefits and taking a greater interest in health and nutrition news.

"This country's obesity crisis has alerted shoppers that they need to take control of their health by taking charge of their diets," said Anne-Marie Roerink, director of research with F.M.I. "In addition, they are increasingly looking to their local supermarkets and other food retailers for effective, long-range solutions." The study examined the shopping habits of 500 consumers nationwide. Thirty-four per cent of consumers surveyed said they believe they are maintaining a healthy diet, while 55% said they are trying "a lot" to eat more healthfully. In addition, 56% said that eating healthfully is a better way to manage illness than taking medications, and 59% claimed they ate healthfully so they can avoid health problems later in life.

5 Schroeder, E. (2004). New Study Suggests Consumers Would Like To Eat Healthier Food. Website: www.bakingbusiness.com

The study showed that consumers seek healthier solutions from manufacturers and retailers. Among the findings, the study found that 46% want their food to offer a greater quantity of nutritiously prepared foods, 45% seek more foods without trans-fatty acids, 40% want more low-fat foods, and 39% want more low-carbohydrate choices.

In what appears to be a good sign for grain-based foods companies developing new products with a health slant, the study showed that consumers are increasingly influenced by the Nutrition Facts panel on food packages. According to the study, 83% of consumers regularly look at the Nutrition Facts chart when buying a product for the first time, while 91% will make a purchasing decision based on this information. About one-fourth have decided not to purchase a product in recent months based on its product labeling information.

The study also found that consumers are interested in other specific product claims, with 63% seeking food promoted as "low-fat" and 62% looking for food promoted as "whole grain." Forty-two per cent of consumers indicated they have purchased foods that claim to reduce their risk of developing heart disease, and 26% have purchased products claiming to reduce the risk of cancer.

(Editor's note: It is even more important to **read the ingredients** – avoiding foods that contain partially hydrogenated fats, preservatives, artificial flavoring, coloring or sweeteners, refined white flour and white sugar or caffeine. You should be able to recognize all the ingredients in real food. *Natural Ovens Bakery uses none of the harmful ingredients listed and you can recognize all of the natural, healthful ingredients.)*

– CHAPTER TWENTY THREE –

WEIGHT WATCHERS

from Jean

I rejoined Weight Watchers November 2001 and have sustained a 40 pound weight loss. I struggled with my weight over most of my adult years, but in my 40s I went into early menopause and gained weight. I am now 51 years old and have radically changed what I eat. I am not fanatical, but have adopted healthier habits that help me stay at a normal weight.

One big help at Weight Watchers was getting so many great ideas for different food choices. Members spoke highly of Natural Ovens' breads. My dad who lives in Manitowoc eats Natural Ovens bread and over the years kept urging me to stop eating white bread and switch. When I rejoined Weight Watchers, I made Natural Ovens bread part of my new life. I was surprised to find that it tasted really good and was more satisfying than other breads. I love the Sunny Millet! Sometimes, when I get hungry, I take two pieces of bread either plain or with some small amount of honey or peanut butter. This helps me avoid binging on chips or crackers. I try to drink eight glasses of water per day. I keep a loaf of Cinnamon Raisin bread at work, in a freezer. If I can not eat breakfast, I reach for that mid day.

I was motivated to lose the weight when I realized that minor health problems were caused by the extra pounds. Achy joints, gastric reflux, back aches, trouble sleeping, all went away after the weight loss. As a nurse, I know that those extra pounds can have a very negative affect on the body. I told myself that only I could make the change and that unlike other times when I lost weight and gained it back, this time, I would need to find good food that I liked and that would fit into my life forever. Now, I always have Natural Ovens bread on hand. I even use it with my hamburgers instead of the white bread buns. Sometimes I buy the bagels and I love the Brainy Bagels.

I still crave certain foods and sometimes I indulge in them. I do not do it real often and I do not tell myself that I can have them as a reward. I try to think of food as fuel and that good fuel makes the body run best. This February I bought a treadmill and so began to exercise regularly, for the first time. I try to get in a walk 3-4 times per week. All of my lifestyle changes were modest. I stopped thinking of a diet as deprivation. I think of it as a permanent change in order to have a healthy life. If I have a week without using the treadmill, or if I have a big dessert, I do not feel guilty. I do however go back to the better choices and so maintain a sense of balance in my life. I think of the changes I have made as the key to a healthier life.

Jean Green Bay, WI

– CHAPTER TWENTY FOUR –

W.W.

from Kathi

I have always maintained a normal, healthy weight by sensible eating, including Natural Ovens Bakery's wonderful products. My husband, however, recently decided to go on Weight Watchers to lose the elusive 10 pounds, but also wants to KEEP it off! He was very successful, since as you must know, WW is a very sensible, slow, healthy weight loss that is easy to maintain with regular smart eating. My tip for you is this: Because we love Natural Ovens' products and have enjoyed them for 25+ years, we definitely wanted to include them and so we were always figuring out the "point value" that each item counts as while using Weight Watchers Winning Point System.

I believe this is the safest diet out there because it's not really a "diet" but good lifestyle eating. Most of Natural Ovens' breads calculate out to be only 1 pt. which is wonderful, because it shows a dieter that they can have a whole sandwich for lunch plus other additions for a healthy meal. The bagels are 3 points (not bad at all) and the muffins are generally 3 points. An example of a healthy breakfast for only 6 points could be: 1 egg (2 points), one muffin (3 points) and a small piece of fruit for 1 point. Natural Ovens' wonderful Great Granola Bars are only 2 points and make a perfect snack. Anyway, you get my point! Enjoy!

Kathi Wright Green Bay, WI

– CHAPTER TWENTY FIVE –

LIFETIME MEMBER

from Sandy

My name is Sandy Greenwood and I lost 120 pounds over 30 years ago. I had always been fighting against weight gain and obviously it hadn't worked. I joined Weight Watchers and over 18 moths lost the 120 pounds. I have stayed in touch with Weight Watchers over the years as a Lifetime Member and watched the program change for the better. I think the trigger was seeing my picture at a wedding and being very unhappy with myself. Over the years I have returned to Weight Watchers when I have put on a few pounds, but have basically kept the weight off all these years. My tastes have definitely changed, for the better.

My way of eating is a lot of vegetables, fruits, whole grains, and of course, when I found them years ago, I only eat Natural Oven's bread and bagels, and oatmeal raisin cookies. I also try to get in 6-8 glasses of water daily. I now dislike fried foods, gravies and such. For the sweet tooth, I eat Natural Ovens' cookies, fruit, and Weight Watchers frozen treats.

I walk two miles every morning with my dog and like to bike ride – things I never did when I was younger. I stay active and keep myself motivated by not liking the way I feel when I put on pounds and try to remember that I don't ever want to go back to my fat life.

I think you have to make your weight loss challenge a way of life and not think of it as a diet, as *diets don't really work.* If you do something regularly, it becomes a habit. It is not always easy, but is definitely worth working for. Natural Ovens' wonderful products, it makes it so much easier.

Sandy Greenwood Sturgeon Bay, WI

– CHAPTER TWENTY SIX –

CAN YOU CHANGE YOUR WAYS?

Here are some good ideas from an excellent article by Carol Cambo.

We are creatures of habit, but change is possible if you have the desire. Motivation for self-improvement stems from caring about yourself. You can do it if you open up to the idea of change and stay focused on the positive end result. Here are tips to affect lasting change.

Know Yourself: When people make behavioral changes without identifying their motivations, behaviors are less likely to stick. Think about what you want to change and why. Write it down in the form of an affirmation and frequently say it out aloud.

Make a Plan: Outline incremental, achievable goals and build in rewards along the way. Measure your progress. "When it comes to losing weight, one of the most effective methods is self-monitoring," says psychologist and weight-loss researcher Daniel Kirschenbaum, PhD, director of the Center for Behavioral Medicine and Sport Psychology in Chicago. "Systematically observing and recording target behaviors, such as reduced calorie and fat intake and increased daily exercise, help you stay on course."

Create an environment for success: If you want to eat better, rid your cupboards of tempting foods and keep healthy snacks on hand. To exercise more, make sure your workout gear is always clean and put it where you can see it. To facilitate self-monitoring, keep a journal and pens readily available.

Swap Bad for Good: Our bad habits fill a need. As you break old patterns you still need a way to meet these needs. Identify what the payoff is for the bad behavior and find a positive way to meet it. If you overeat when you're tired or stressed out, try napping, meditating, or going for a walk instead. If you order high-calorie takeout to save time, prepare a healthy meal but use paper plates to cut down on cleanup. Or learn what you can order that won't throw you off track.

Join Forces: Numerous studies have shown that if you partner up with one or more people with similar goals, you're more likely to achieve them. Look for others to get involved, such as enlisting a friend for regular walks or trips to the gym.

Strategize for Relapses: If you have a plan for how to deal with failure, you'll spend less negative energy on the relapse and be able to get back on track.

– CHAPTER TWENTY SEVEN –

MORE WEIGHT WATCHERS

from Karen

I have been overweight to obese since a toddler. Four years ago this November, I had some health struggles and a friend who was losing weight for her health. It really brought it home to me that I needed to lose weight or become diabetic or worse. I wanted to still have choices and control of my food (I love to cook and enjoy food immensely.) So, I followed my friend into Weight Watchers (after many attempts at losing, I had vowed never to join a group). In the next 14 months, I lost 75 pounds and have stayed at this weight for 2.5 years. Totally unheard of for me and my history! My nuclear and extended family were so shocked they all tried it too – we lost a total of 350 pounds!

So, my secrets? First, change the way you think about this process – *diet* is a negative word, filled with self-denial and bad feelings. Use the Weight Watchers "program" and you will find lots of recipes and freedom of choice. I found over time, that I really like my vegetables and fruits and when I could stay within my "points" range it was such a boost to my self-esteem.

Second, use the high fiber/low calorie/low fat directive when making most of your food choices and you will stay on track better. That's why I am ordering Natural Ovens bread online. Seems a little crazy, but I can't get such healthy choices here in Saginaw, MI. In general, I find that increasing fiber creates fullness and satiety very well – and Natural Ovens has lots of choices that do that.

Third, I was a dedicated couch potato. I just started walking about half an hour each day and that really boosted the weight loss. As the weight came off, I was more active throughout the day and that same half hour walk plus just doing my work actively, keeps the weight off. (I also still count my points daily – discipline now plays a role that I can accept once I truly know I can DO this!) I also found I could eat more as my metabolism got a boost – I am shocked at how much I eat, and NEED to eat to keep me going.

My continual motivation is that I don't ever want to be that fat, tired, unhappy person again—and I don't want to inflict her on my family either! Also, my health improved so significantly that I am off some of my meds and my doctor can't say enough about how I have done what he wants for so many other patients. By the way, I am 56 and quite active now—so much so that I took the Christian Education position at my church 2 years ago and run with the children in all our programs with ease!

My family was very supportive of my effort—even from long distance. When they actually saw me, they didn't recognize me. So, since I was transformed they went for it too-- and it worked, but some of them have regained some of the weight. (They were dieting and went back to old habits.) I continue to encourage them.

I also wanted to share that I work in a medical office and the PA lost 60 pounds and kept if off for years. More recently, the nurse lost 52, the receptionist lost 25, the biller lost 30 and I lost 75—all on Weight Watchers. We posted our before pictures on a board at the check out desk titled "while you are weighting" and many patients want to talk about our loss and some have done it too.

Karen Saginaw, MI

– CHAPTER TWENTY EIGHT –

OUTGROWN

from Barb Killen

I began Weight Watchers in January of 1998 and lost 60 pounds in 9 months which I have kept off since then. I was motivated to begin because I had "outgrown" all my clothes and decided they were going to be smaller not larger.

I never thought of it as dieting but rather as a new way of living. I began eating breakfast, drinking more water, and exercising daily. To me it really is very basic but I needed the support of others and the weekly weigh-ins to keep me honest. I still attend meetings to keep me on track. If I slip a little now and then I get re-energized and back to eating healthy and within my limits.

I have joined Curves to give myself a change in exercise routine even though I have a treadmill and elliptical machine at home. The variety keeps me from getting bored and helps use all different muscles. I work out 60 minutes daily.

I eat Natural Ovens' breads, bagels and granola bars that are low in points, high in fiber, and satisfy my hunger. I eat a minimum of 5 fruits and vegetables a day. With that in mind, each day I find myself snacking on grapes, apples, etc. rather than chips and cookies. In the past I had a difficult time avoiding the candy bars at the check out lane and now I crave cherries, bananas, peaches—all the wonderful fresh fruits in the summer!

I do keep a journal of what I eat each day. I found it too easy to overeat if I didn't actually stop and think about what I was putting in my mouth. The rewards of weight loss have been great for me. I feel better, sleep better, have much more energy, and now can buy clothes I like instead of always looking for something just to cover up my bulging middle.

In my opinion there is no magic solution or pill that will make it easy. It is just the *basics of eating smaller portions,* eating a well balanced diet and exercising that makes it work. These all have to be daily just like brushing your teeth and taking a shower. You just do it! Not just until you reach your weight goal but for the rest of your life.

Barb Killen

– CHAPTER TWENTY NINE –

THE GAIN GAME[6]

Getting older sure can hit you where it hurts: your waistline. Whether you're in your twenties, thirties, or forties, you've probably noticed that with every passing decade it gets tougher to stay (or get) slim. In fact, maybe your diet hasn't changed at all, but your pants are getting tighter. Or shedding a few pounds was a breeze in the past, but now it's downright impossible. And the gain pain isn't just cosmetic: We've known for some time that obesity is linked to health conditions like diabetes, hypertension, heart disease, and some cancers, but researchers are now connecting being overweight directly to life span. One study found that people who became obese by age 40 lose, on average, seven years of their life. So if you think you're too young to worry about a few extra pounds, or too old to turn back the clock, you're not. With the right strategy, you can gain years, lose pounds, and get healthy at every decade — starting now.

At any age it is vitally important that you drink filtered water (1 oz for each 2 lbs) and get about 2,000 mg of vitamin D from the sun or by supplement.

In your 20s

Great news for your diet: In your twenties, your metabolic rate remains relatively high, meaning you're still burning calories with ease. On the downside, while you might not see any fat building up on your hips, it is starting to

6 Vitetta-Miller, R. (2003). The Gain Game. Weight Watchers Magazine

accumulate around your internal organs and under the skin. So while skipping exercise and eating poorly may seem like no big deal, research says otherwise: In addition to weight gain, your belly fat could be setting you up for heart disease, high blood pressure, and diabetes down the line.

And let's not forget osteoporosis. What you may not realize is that even at age 20 your bones aren't fully formed — they continue to strengthen through your late twenties. So short-change your diet of dark leafy green vegetables now and you may be compromising the future health and well-being of your bones.

Now is also the time to start consuming a health-promoting diet that's rich in whole grains; fruits; vegetables; high-quality, lean protein (such as skinless chicken, turkey, fish, shellfish, eggs, and soy); and heart-healthy fats (such as fish, olives and olive oils, seeds, nuts and nut oils). *Be careful to avoid soda, sugar and white flour, junk foods, and artificially colored, sweetened, and flavored foods.*

And when it comes to exercise, this is the decade to flaunt it. You've still got the time and the energy to create a fitness routine that will become a natural part of your life for years to come. Try thinking of your fitness plan the way you think of your 401K: Invest now and you'll reap the benefits later. And whatever activity you choose, be sure to exercise for at least 30 minutes most days of the week.

In your 30s

Hormone levels (estrogen and progesterone) gradually begin falling now. This is important because estrogen affects appetite — when estrogen levels are high, appetite drops;

when estrogen is low (right before your menstrual cycle), appetite increases. Metabolism also starts to slow down when you hit your thirties. According to Dan Benardot, PhD, co director of the Laboratory for Elite Athletic Performance at Georgia State University in Athens, "Metabolism declines by two percent each decade after the age of 30 — so, if you eat what you always ate and your metabolism is slower, guess what? You're going to gain weight." He adds, "At the same time, there is a shift away from lean body mass and a shift toward fat mass. This shift in body composition means that most of the weight we gain is fat, not muscle."

When it comes to your diet, practice reverse psychology: Don't eat more, but do eat more often. Eating regularly stimulates an increase in metabolism, so increase the number of times you eat each day, starting with breakfast, to jump-start your metabolism. "Spread nutritious meals and snacks throughout the day so you're eating about every three hours," recommends Katherine Tallmadge, spokesperson for the American Dietetic Association.

While a hectic schedule — juggling work and family demands or a busy social calendar — may have you reaching for frequent java jolts, have a glass of water instead and resist the temptation — for your health and your weight. It's a misconception that caffeine and other stimulants can spur weight loss. Too much caffeine can actually cause a fast rise in blood sugar, followed by a fast drop — which can send hunger signals to your brain. Caffeine can also interfere with your body's absorption of calcium, which can lead to osteoporosis as you age. But there's no need to blacklist your local

Starbucks — just curb your caffeine allotment by sticking to an A.M. cup only, or trying the new "light" coffees available now in supermarkets — they're made with half the caffeine of regular coffee.

Exercise is the best way to beat the gain in your thirties. Muscle revs up metabolism and extra muscle means extra calories burned — even when your body is at rest. Maintain an exercise routine or accelerate your current program (strive for at least 30 minutes of cardio at least five days per week and strength train at least two times per week). "Strength training keeps muscles strong as you age, combating the inevitable shift in your body composition from muscle to fat," says Benardot. But combining strength training with a cardio routine is key, since aerobic exercise contributes to your cardiovascular health.

In your 40s

In this decade, unless you work out with weights, you're continuing to lose muscle mass, and your metabolism is slowing down. Fat is more easily stored — particularly in your midsection (tummy). Your hormone levels drop further, meaning you're losing the heart-protective effects of estrogen. And you face an increased risk of heart disease, high blood pressure, and diabetes. Since diet is the single biggest predictor of all three diseases, the choices you make now can have a major impact on your future health.

Although the average age of menopause is 51, some women will have symptoms of peri-menopause (the precursor to menopause) during this decade, says Shari Lieberman, PhD, a clinical nutritionist and menopause researcher in New York City. "Menopause is a major hormonal event in women, and it alone will significantly affect your metabolic rate," says Lieberman.

Keep your diet lean and mean in your forties — eliminate empty calories and fill up on low-calorie fruits, vegetables, and whole grains. You'll get a jump on preventing heart disease and other middle-age health woes.

Another reason to go lean? A healthy diet may spell menopause relief. A study in the *Journal of Obstetrics and Gynecology* found that obesity may predispose women to hot flashes during menopause. Women in the study with a body mass index (BMI) greater than 30 were more likely to report moderate to severe hot flashes than those who had a BMI less than 25.

More good news? Build on your exercise and a cardio workout — the first prevents bone loss, and the second helps you gain muscle mass, which will rev up your metabolism and help you burn calories more effectively," says Dr. Lieberman.

Try mountain biking (a great workout for you and your honey), power walking, or a tougher workout like a Spinning or a kick-boxing class. And whatever you do, do it daily — or at least five days a week, for maximum results.

This article is reprinted from Weight Watchers Magazine, May/June 2003.

— CHAPTER THIRTY —

OUTSIDE THE BOX

from Grace

Let me first say that my husband and I discovered Natural Ovens bread over ten years ago. When it comes to bread, we have been enjoying it almost exclusively, having introduced it to friends and family along the way. Needless to say, it is a staple in our diet, along with Great Granola and Paul's Oats as healthy supplements.

We are both 65 years old, and though we are not on a specific weight-loss regimen, we are mindful of the need to practice good nutrition. Like so many, we do well in some instances, and not so well in others. Thanks to Natural Ovens, however, these products have provided motivation for improvement, and emphasized the necessity of good nutrition.

Some years ago, we stopped eating traditional breakfasts of eggs, bacon, pancakes/waffles, etc. due to the new knowledge on the dangers of cholesterol. After developing lactose intolerance approximately nine years ago, cold cereals were no longer a good option. Consequently, we began eating breakfast limited to only fresh fruit consisting of a citrus fruit, an apple, a pear, and a banana. This is supplemented with other varieties in season. (Editor's note: Almond Milk, Rice or Soy Milk are great with Great Granola for a wonderfully sustaining breakfast.)

My husband prepares the fruit every day, slicing into wedges, coring, and serving ready-to-eat. He accompanies the fruit with Natural Ovens toast; no butter. (No toast for me at this meal.) My husband has three slices in the morning, and as much as two at lunch and two at supper (mostly toasted) with no resulting weight gain. However, my system will not tolerate near that amount of bread without weight gain, proving that it is vital that we know our body limitations. (Editor's note: The new Golden Crunch Bread, 100% Whole Grain, Original Lo Carb and Sunny Millet Breads are all low on the glycemic index and won't cause the weight gain.)

Though somewhat unconventional, the following are some cooking habits that have contributed to healthier meals. Here are just a few ideas that I would like to share. I will preface these ideas by saying that you must be willing to think "outside the box."

1. When cooking stew, or any recipe which requires a thickening agent, as a substitute for white unbleached flour or cornstarch, I use plain, raw oatmeal. Through the cooking process, oatmeal takes on the flavor of the recipe be it a main dish, gravies, sauces, or any recipe requiring thickening.

2. Rather than purchasing prepared croutons, I toast Natural Ovens bread of any variety. Cut into cubes and place in a bowl, spraying with fat-free pan spray of personal choice, making sure all cubes are lightly coated. Sprinkle spices of preference such as oregano and basil for Italian spiced croutons. Variety is only limited to your creativity and taste buds. Bake in oven at 350-375 just long enough to

reach the right degree of crunchiness. The end result is not only tasty and healthy, but a fraction of the cost of prepared croutons.

3. We don't purchase jellies or jams. My husband thinly slices fresh fruits such as mangos, peaches, strawberries, bananas, or kiwi. Simply stack on Natural Ovens bread of any variety to create a virgin "jam" containing only nature's ingredients. Ripe bananas will also spread nicely.

4. Cubed, Natural Ovens Happiness Bread makes an excellent bread pudding using cholesterol-free egg product, and crystalline fructose as a natural sweetener.

Grace Prescott, AZ

– CHAPTER THIRTY ONE –

INSPIRATION

from Leah

Being 30 and after having our second child, my husband and I knew we were done having children. It was time to start focusing on myself again. I wanted to look the way I looked 5 years ago–pre children. One of the changes I decided to make in my life was to learn how to eat healthier and lose weight. I have never been on a professional weight loss management program, but my friend Patty had joined Weight Watchers and had great success…she was my inspiration.

I'm never hungry and have learned to choose high fiber, low calorie and low fat choices which fill me up and keep me satisfied. Considering this a lifestyle change and not a diet–my number one goal was to learn to eat healthier and to maximize what I am putting in my mouth. Being a huge fan of bread, I learned to eat all the Natural Ovens Bakery products.

I have learned so much like eating 100% Whole Grain and high fiber with the Flax and Omega-3. My favorite products are the Brainy Bagel and the Hunger Filler Bread. I have lost over 30 pounds by learning to eat correctly and controlling portion sizes, I am now back in a size 6 and am happy to report it is thanks to Natural Ovens Bakery and Weight Watchers. Thank you Natural Ovens Bakery!

Leah

– CHAPTER THIRTY TWO –

THE OKINAWA PLAN

from Tina

My best friend joined Weight Watchers in January of 2001. I decided to join too, so people wouldn't know me as "that skinny girl's fat friend". It took less than six months to lose 22 pounds and reach my goal weight. I have kept that weight off even though I had a baby in 2003.

Besides the grace of God, there are two primary reasons for this. The first is that I've made nutrition a hobby. I read everything I can find regarding diet and nutrition – including Natural Ovens' newsletters in every loaf of bread! I've read at least four books, subscribed to three magazines, and I even saw *Super Size Me!* Most influential has been the *Okinawa Program* by Willcox, Willcox, and Suzuki. That book explained with clarity and details the importance of a healthy heart and blood vessels, good and bad cholesterol, and the effects of diet on these things. They attribute most of the fact that Okinawans have 80% fewer heart attacks than Americans to the junk we eat. This book was the first I had ever heard about trans fat. We are literally poisoning ourselves with trans fat and refined carbohydrates! It still appalls me how little coverage this gets even in so-called fitness media. But as Barbara and Paul, owners of Natural Ovens Bakery know, big money is involved in keeping it quiet.

This new knowledge translated into some new habits regarding food. If the ingredients include hydrogenated oil (in any quantity), I don't buy it! This step alone has huge implications, because everything in a box contains hydrogenated oil. What is left are whole, unprocessed foods that are high in fiber and nutrition, but low in salt, chemicals, and preservatives: fresh and frozen fruits and vegetables, whole grain rice, millet, anything made by Natural Ovens Bakery, unprocessed chicken, salmon, or tuna, natural almond or peanut butter and soy products, and most organic foods. In addition to limiting processed foods at the supermarket, I almost never eat fast food unless it is a salad (with the dressing on the side).

In addition to eliminating trans fats, I've been trying to work up to the 7-13 vegetable and 2-4 fruit servings The Okinawa Plan recommends. I can't say enough about vegetables. They're low in calories and loaded with nutrition. If you make vegetables half your meal, there's just no room for a lot of calorie-dense foods. I do have some treats like pizza and the occasional chocolate malt, but I try to limit high-calorie treats to once per week. This keeps me from bringing on forbidden foods.

The second reason for my maintenance has been a willingness to be accountable when necessary by writing down what I eat and seeking group support. Even without restrictions, I was able to keep my pregnancy weight gain under 30 pounds just by writing everything down – it prevented mindless nibbling. Although I'm no longer at Weight Watchers, I am attending a program at my church called First Place. This group keeps me accountable but places more emphasis on God's balance between spiritual, emotional, physical, and social health.

I also eat real salad dressing, but I limit my portions by the fork-dipping rather than pouring it on. Extra Virgin Olive Oil is a healthy source of mono-saturated fat and is digested slower than fat-free dressing, which is mostly corn syrup, so it keeps blood sugar more even. My diet is probably higher in fat than most experts recommend because I often eat meat alternatives like natural peanut butter, soy, and eggs. These foods are easier on my polycystic kidneys because they are lower in protein, but they are higher in fat than lean meat.

I drink 60-90 oz of water everyday, plus 20-40 oz of decaf coffee. I usually flavor my water with lemon juice or I mix 1 part 100% fruit juice to 3 or 4 parts water. If I'm in the mood for something fizzy, I use flavored seltzer instead of plain water. I never drink soda or full-strength juice. They're just too sweet.

I walk and jog with my dog 3-4 days per week and enjoy a nice, long stretch afterward. I want to go to the YMCA and lift weights twice per week because I know from experience that the more muscle I have, the more I can eat, but I've had a hard time since my son was born with the 40 minutes of driving time.

As a wife and mom, I am responsible for preparing healthy food for my family. I also need to set a good example for my son to follow. That keeps me motivated. I seem to have done okay. My 16-month-old's favorite foods are peas, broccoli and bananas. I hope this letter is helpful and thank you for the opportunity to share and for your wonderful Natural Ovens products.

Tina Omro, WI

– CHAPTER THIRTY THREE –

STOMACH PROBLEMS

from Rachael

I just wanted to let you know how much I love Natural Ovens' breads and bagels. Your Golden Crunch Bagel with only 7 grams of net carbs has actually lowered my morning insulin dosage!!! I have had diabetes for 12 years and in the past few have eaten Natural Ovens' breads with many benefits that I never thought could happen since being diabetic for numerous years.

I had stomach problems a lot, irregular and always hungry. Natural Ovens' products have rid all of these problems and on top of that, supply many nutrients and vitamins I just wouldn't get if I didn't eat these breads. My insulin needs have lessened because the products have so much natural fiber which slows the absorption of glucose in my blood, thus I don't need such high doses of the insulin when I eat Natural Ovens' bread.

Thanks so much and please keep coming out with low carb products. I buy them like crazy!

Rachael

– CHAPTER THIRTY FOUR –

FOODIE

from Linda

Let me begin by explaining that I am a real Foodie. Except for liver, I have not met a food I do not like. I owe a lot of that to the way I ate as a child. I was raised by a mother who made all our bread throwing last night's vegetable water in for extra nutrition, and by a mother who served us breakfast as a family every morning and supper each evening. She is a frugal woman, so her meals included garden grown produce, home-canned vegetables and relishes, and little meat. She also kept our menus varied and interesting and instilled my confidence around the kitchen.

I never had problems with my weight until I was 21, and after a particularly stressful first year of teaching dropped to 135 pounds. (I am 5'11"). My body started going into starvation mode – I started missing my period, I spent more and more time sleeping and depressed. Worse yet, I believe that year significantly served to slow my metabolism.

Around February of 2001, being 37 years old, I came to the realization that I did not like my body and that two options were open to me: resolve to love myself within that body, or lose the weight. At that point I was 231 pounds and, although others would not classify me as grossly obese, I was beyond feeling attractive. – I was big.

I started trying to lose weight on my own using common sense: water, walk, portion control and lots of nonfood rewards. Progress was slow and by May I had lost only 5 pounds. One May night I was sitting with some of my neighbors when one of them asked if I would like to join her in trying out Weight Watchers. She had pirated the book form a girl at work and we could do it together. That's when the weight started coming off. I applied that same patient determination that had endured the 2.5 months-5 pounds, but now I was losing two or three pounds a week!

Weight Watchers works for me. Because I enjoy cooking, points are easy to figure. I find it fairly easy to figure points in my head based on what I know is in a recipe (e.g. what makes risotto creamy is not actual cream, but Arborio rice). I have to be bold, because ordering at a restaurant comes with a list of substitutions, omissions and instructions. Another reason it works for me is that I have such a varied pallet: it is satisfying to me to end a meal with a sorbet rather than a flourless chocolate torte.

I will say that there were times I would slip into self pity: "how can he get away with eating that and I can't even let it cross my mind?" One of the most powerful lessons came when I learned that a good friend of mine was diagnosed with diabetes. I found myself feeling sorry for him that his whole life would now have to change. Hello!?! It sunk in – just like the diabetic (or the alcoholic or the child with PKU etc.) I had a condition that was going to kill me if I did not make some life-long changes. Framed in that, I bless the fact that something forced me to eat the way I should so that I could have the quality of life I have: I have the energy of someone 10 years my junior, I don't get sick often and when I get sick it does not last long, I look great in my clothes, the aches in my knees are gone, my asthma is gone, and my self-confidence has sky-rocketed.

Life changes do not end at counting points. By December of 2001 I had reached my goal weight of 170. I knew that this weight was acceptable to me, but weight was more than numbers on a scale. The point now was to eat right and live right. I knew by now this diet didn't fix my problem, my problem would last my whole life. The diet was there to maintain what I had come to expect out of life. The weight loss continued and by New Year's Eve I was down to 160. That was the evening my friend Pat asked me if he could train me. I balked at the idea. I did not see myself as an athlete and really did not relish the thought of exercise. I decided another discipline couldn't hurt – so I gave it a try. Twice a week I would meet with him (he volunteered his services – another blessing) and we would work with weights and setting up my own fitness goals.

Another 10 pounds and a year and a half later – I ran the Chicago Marathon in 4:33:27 – a 40 year old birthday present to myself. I continue running and working with weights and floor exercises to help with the days when my will power falters. I lost 80 pounds in all, but I gained so much more – my life. Here are tips that I give others when they ask.

I have literally become a bread snob who knows the difference between multi grain and whole grain. And I am totally spoiled by only charging myself one point for two slices of Natural Ovens Bakery breads.

At a barbecue – forgo the bun. Make your plate one big salad instead – using the condiments and the meat.

Learn your appetite suppressors. Licorice or coffee help me close a dinner so that I do not need dessert – so I carry licorice in my purse when I go out. Mint gum helps me not snack on cheese (my toughest temptation).

Bring your lunch to work. Use Natural Ovens' bread – really.

At work, always keep a healthy snack available for when you need an option for that treat one of your coworkers brought in.

Give yourself a chance to experiment with food in your own kitchen. It will not always turn out, but you will come to understand it better.

Nothing tastes as good as thin feels.

Take dietary supplements.

Drink water, but not too much. Americans have gone overboard on their water (so what's new?!). I found I only need 6 cups a day from a formula I read in Runner's World Magazine.

Get the bad food out of the house!

Move your body. Park far and walk. Stairs, not escalators. Walk, don't ride. Dance.

At restaurants:

Ask them not to leave the bread basket on the table.

Order light white fish, chicken or ostrich prepared by grilling or baking and served with a fresh sauce. Careful – fish is often served in a drawn butter. Remember salmon and Tuna are fatty (good fat – but fat you still have to burn).

When you order something that is higher in fat than makes you comfortable, ask for a take home container to be brought at the same time as your meal. Promptly unload half your plate into the container and place it beneath your seat. You are less inclined to eat it if you would be seen eating out of a doggie bag.

Order any questionable dressings or sauces on the side. Before you take a bite of the salad or meat – dip your fork into the sauce.

Don't be fooled. All salads are not created equal. It is better to order a broth soup than a salad made from iceberg lettuce (which has absolutely no nutritional value apart from filler and water).

Careful with the alcohol – carbs apart – it does lower your self control.

Linda Mathematics Teacher

– CHAPTER THIRTY FIVE –

DIABETIC

from Carmen

Three years ago I was diagnosed diabetic. I was 51 years old, and grossly obese. The doctor was ready to put me on meds, but I begged for a three month reprieve to see if I could make a significant change on my own. I got nutritional counseling, and the okay for a strenuous walking plan. My two major hurdles would be chocolate and bread.

I quit chocolate cold turkey. Don't laugh! It was bad. I was totally dependent on the two things. Bread was another story. I couldn't give it up. A month into my self devised plan, I found Natural Ovens breads. The angels sang the Hallelujah Chorus that day! I can have as many as 6 slices a day if I'm feeling needy. My favorites are Multi Grain, Hunger Filler and the Soft Wheat. My husband is a hard working construction superintendent and the breads are fabulous for him, too.

Back to the results of the first three months: My A1C was 6.7, cholesterol and triglycerides were down, and I dropped a dress size. To date, I am still on the same program, still losing (5 dress sizes, 1 1/2 shoe sizes, smaller hats, etc!), feel fabulous, and have made myself proud. I eat three nutritionally balanced meals a day, and three to four snacks. My friends don't get it: they think all I do it eat! I use chicken, fish, ground turkey, fresh vegetables (raw or cooked), fresh fruits, and whole grains. I cook from scratch. That's important! Once you make the change, your body insists on staying with it. You feel good, you look good, your hair and skin improves, stamina is up, and you are able to cope with whatever life throws you in a much more effective manner.

I have a visualization trick that helped me tremendously from day 1: I envision anything made of white flour as "cotton candy"; YUCK! It takes away my desire for white flour products, and other undesirable "treats". I am continuing my lifestyle change forever. I will reach my goal about next spring, and will hopefully celebrate with a new wardrobe. I have to tell you that without Natural Ovens' breads (and bagels, and cookies...), I don't think that I would have done well. I travel with Natural Ovens breads! I take my own sandwiches to luncheons. I don't care what people think, and if they give me grief, I show them a before picture and tell them to try my plan. To date, I am controlling my diabetes with diet and exercise, and have impressed my doctors, nutritionist, and friends! Thanks Natural Ovens!

Most sincerely,

Carmen

– CHAPTER THIRTY SIX –

NOT AGAIN

from Katherine

I lost 50 pounds two years ago with Weight Watchers, and am happy to share some of the details of what has worked for me. I am in total agreement, by the way, with the statement that there are many ways to LOSE the weight. The true challenge is keeping it off over time! I've lost the same weight twice, and have definitely learned a few tings this time around. I will NOT lose this weight again!

I had gained my weight gradually: 10 pounds in high school, 10 pounds in college, 10 pounds in law school, and 10 pounds working long hours in my first job after law school. I joined Weight Watchers in 1987, and lost nearly 50 pounds by following their program. At that time, it was fairly rigid, and did not place much emphasis on exercise. After I reached my goal, I stopped journaling my food, stopped attending meetings and stopped weighing myself. Not surprisingly, within a few years, I'd put most of the weight back on. I got married (to a man who eats whatever he wants and never gains a pound, the bum!), had a child, and reached my all time high weight of 187 (I am 5'8").

During the summer of 2002, we visited one of my best friends from college and her family in San Francisco. Three separate things on that trip combined to form my weight loss "trigger": a) it struck me that my friend is exactly my height and looked exactly the same as she did in college, while I was so much heavier and looked so much older; b) her then 4-year-old daughter, at a point when we were alone together, looked at me and said "You know, you're really fat!"; and c) at one point, all seven of us (four adults and three kids in car seats) were trying to fit into their minivan. I tried to sit in the middle seat between two of the car seats, but could not jam my large rear end into the space! Both my friend and my husband easily could. Upon returning home, I immediately destroyed all the pictures from that trip. Fortunately, my friend sent me one that she had taken. I say fortunately, because that has become my "before" picture now that I've lost the weight!

I had been putting off going back to Weight Watchers, figuring that I knew what to do, and didn't need to pay them to weigh me, but somehow, I never did it! Well, after that trip, I realized that by not going back to a structure that had worked for me, I was making a choice to remain heavy, unhappy, and unhealthy.

What worked for me before worked again. Weight Watchers is a great program that emphasizes healthy foods, controlled portions, and moderate exercise. I began journaling my food, reading food labels, watching portion sizes, and walking for exercise regularly. I drank

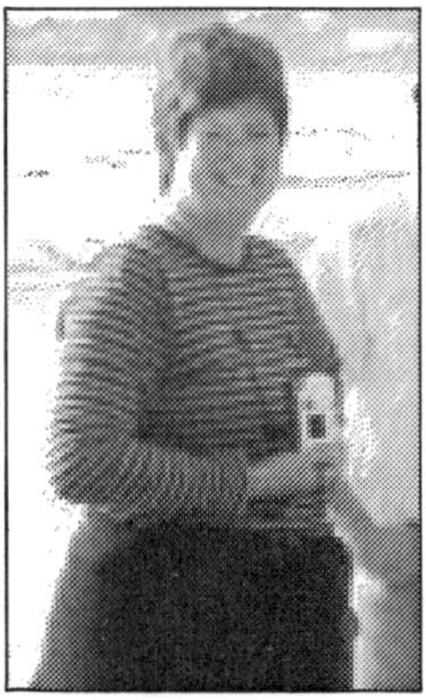

Katherine's "before" photo

at least 64 oz. of water each day. One of the products I relied on the most was Natural Ovens' Sunny Millet bread. Two slices with a tablespoon of peanut butter, and whatever fruit looks good in the market, are STILL my breakfast of choice! I am a volume eater...I like to feel full. Well, on Weight Watchers, that means vegetables! I will steam a whole head of broccoli, and eat most of it myself. My husband (who does most of the cooking—lucky me!) knows that he needs to make the salad bowl twice as big as in the "old days". I treat myself to pricier vegetables I love (like artichokes and snow peas), knowing that I am still spending less than I was on the less healthy things I was filling up on, like fried rice, or fettuccine alfredo.

After losing 10 pounds, I felt so much better, and the better I felt, the more activities I felt like doing. I started running a little, alternating with walking (I had never been able to run before, because my knees hurt too badly.) When I was finally running more than I was walking (it took about six months), I signed up for an 8K (5 mile) race with my husband. He promised to stick with me, even though he is a stronger runner. The feeling of accomplish-

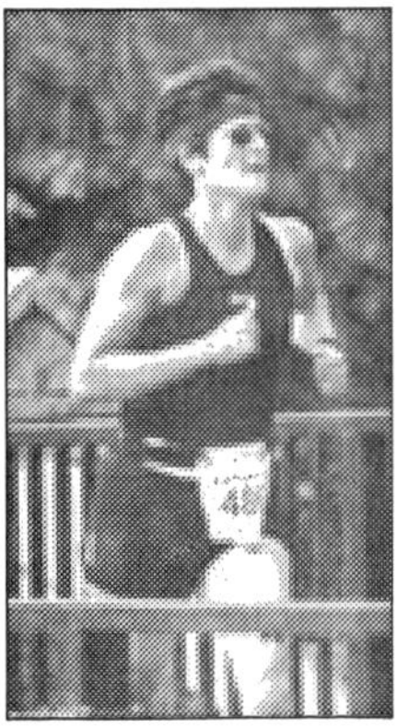

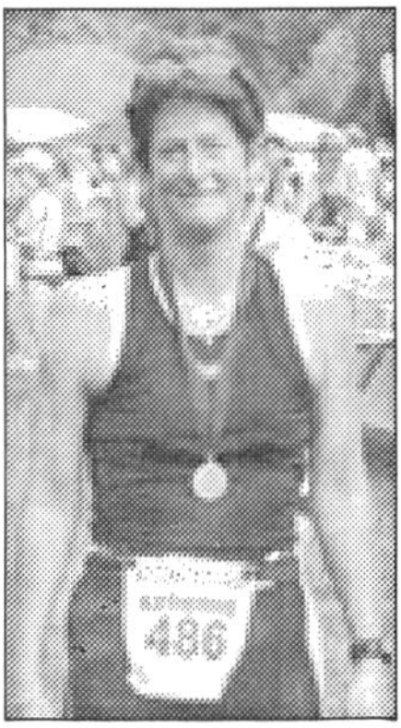

Katherine's "after" photos

ment coming across that finish line was something I could not have imagined! Little did I know that it would be the first of many such achievements. I've now completed two 8Ks, two 10Ks, five or six 5Ks, a metric century (62 miles) bike ride, and this past weekend, I completed my first triathlon (1/2 mile swim, 14.5 mile bike and 5K run). I had a ball doing it, and ended up finishing in the top third of the 149 women in my age group (45-49), and in the top 40% of all participants. My post-triathlon picture is now my official "after" shot, and I look forward to doing longer distances as my training allows!

If you'd told me two years ago that I'd be doing a triathlon, I'd have called you crazy! However, the exercise, while allowing me to eat more than I'd otherwise be able to, is not a "free ride". I still journal my food (which is a pain, but such a small thing when weighed against the way I look and feel now), attend Weight Watcher meetings regularly, and drink lots of water.

My tastes have changed in some regards. Fried foods simply do not taste as good as they used to. I still enjoy red meat, but in smaller quantities now, as I think the fat just overwhelms my system! I still love salty, crunchy snacks, but will generally reach for reduced-fat crackers or rice cakes instead of chips or cheese puffs! Of course, Natural Ovens' products continue to play a big part in my eating plan. I eat at least two servings of your breads a day, and treat myself to your bagels or muffins once a month or so. I love Natural Ovens' commitment to high fiber and no trans fats.

On the subject of "treats", I think one of the components of successful maintenance is recognizing that no food is totally "evil" or even off-limits. As long as I work it into my food plan for the day, I will have a piece of birthday cake, or a slice of pizza, or an ice cream cone. It really is human nature that as soon as you say you can't have a certain food; it gains a weird power over you! I know that I can continue to enjoy anything I want…in moderation.

Three things keep me motivated. First, I want to model good eating and overall good health for my daughter who is now five. She deserves to grow up with a healthy, thin and active mom! Second, I just FEEL so much better at this weight, and I am so enjoying what my fit body allows me to accomplish athletically, and in day-to day living. Lastly, I love being able to have just one set of clothes in the closet rather than a range of sizes to cover fluctuating weights. Keeping weight off is a continuing project, but I am at a stage now (it took nearly a year) where I know what I have to do, don't feel deprived, and am quite certain that I will never have to lose that 50 pounds again!

Katherine Chicago, IL

– CHAPTER THIRTY SEVEN –

THE CABBAGE SOUP DIET

Many of the stories you just read had two things in common. Those two things were increased exercise and a change in lifestyle by choosing healthy eating over hydrogenated fats, white flour, and sugars. We would like to share some helpful hints we have accumulated over the years. Enjoy and good luck on your journey to a healthier life.

Paul & Barbara Stitt
Owners – Natural Ovens Bakery

Also called "The Dolly Parton diet," for reasons that are shrouded in mystery, this 7-day diet really does work--in the short term, anyway. And there's a great purity to it--especially in the summertime when it's wonderfully refreshing served ice cold. Ingredient proportions can be varied according to your likes and dislikes. Please read to the end of the recipe where you'll find testimony and great ideas regarding the diet from readers. Hunger Filler Bread, Golden Crunch Bread, Great Granola Cereal, and C and D Plus are available in your favorite super market in the Midwest or at www.naturalovens.com – or call 1-800-772-0730.

Cabbage Soup recipe

1 head cabbage, shredded or chopped

2 large onions, chopped

16-28 ounces canned tomatoes, chopped

2 red or orange bell peppers

4 stalks celery

1-2 package dry onion soup mix or
3T chicken flavor – in powder form found
in Natural Foods Sections...

Black pepper

Any fresh herb(s) of your choice, chopped.
Use lots

1 small turnip, if you can find it.
It adds a wonderful flavor

6 carrots, sliced

1/2 pound green beans, sliced on diagonal

1/4 cup balsamic vinegar (optional)

Put all vegetables in a big pot and cover with water. Bring to a boil, stir in the soup mix (if desired), and boil gently for 10 minutes. Cover, reduce heat, and simmer until all the vegetables are soft. Stir in the black pepper and chopped herbs (saving some for garnish). Serves 6-8.

Serve with Whole Grain Toast

Eat as much of the soup as you like, as often as you like. Take a B-complex and a half-teaspoon of C & D Plus (from Natural Ovens Bakery) three times a day. Drink as much water and herbal teas as you like – at least 8 glasses daily..

Here's what else you can eat, and when:

DAY 1: All fruits except bananas. 1 slice of Natural Ovens Hunger Filler Bread, 100% Whole Grain, Sunny Millet or Golden Crunch Bread with each bowl of cabbage soup...beginning when you feel hungry and all the soup you want for the rest of the day.

DAY 2: Any vegetables, raw or cooked. All the cabbage soup you want and 1-3 slices of Golden Crunch or Hunger Filler Bread and 8 glasses of water.

DAY 3: Fresh fruit, melon, berries for breakfast and all the soup you want all day. 8 glasses of water.

DAY 4: 1 Banana with a small bowl of Great Granola with almond or soy milk for breakfast. All the cabbage soup you want for the rest of the day. Have 1 slice of Natural Ovens Golden Crunch bread with 2 of the bowls of soup. 8 glasses of water

DAY 5: 1/2 cup of Great Granola for breakfast, a small bowl of cabbage soup plus 3-4 oz. skinless chicken or fish with fresh tomatoes for lunch. Have all the cabbage soup you want and 1 slice of Golden Crunch or 100% Whole Grain bread with each of 2 of the bowls for the remainder of the day. 8 glasses of water throughout the day.

DAY 6: Fresh sliced orange and two slices of Golden Crunch toast for breakfast. Have 3 or 4 oz. skinless chicken or fish with steamed vegetables for brunch or lunch. Eat all the Cabbage soup you want for the rest of the day. Remember the water!

DAY 7: Great Granola with raspberries or blue berries for breakfast, (always have small portions which will be satisfying but without the stuffed feeling) – A cup of soup, Brown rice, vegetables, and unsweetened fruit juice for lunch and all the cabbage soup you want for rest of the day. You should lose 7 to 10 pounds in the 7 days – and feel wonderfully good energy.

If more weight loss is needed, eat normally of fresh fruits, vegetables, whole grains, legumes, brown rice, 1 or 2 eggs, 4-oz. of fish or chicken a day (if not vegetarian), salads etc. then repeat the cabbage soup diet every other week...until you are the weight you desire. If 4 or 5 pounds creep back, simply do the diet for several days and it will be gone. You will find that you no longer want to overeat and stretch your stomach again. Enjoy!

TESTIMONY!

If you're interested in going gourmet AND losing weight, try the following suggestions, recommended by Bobbi B. from California: "To make the soup not so impossible to eat three times a day; try making the first batch with red onions, red cabbage and red bell peppers, leave it chunky like a minestrone. The second batch make with yellow onions, green cabbage & green bells (I left out the tomatoes in second batch) and purée it. The taste and texture change makes it so much more palatable. Hey! I lost 10 lbs. in 7 days, I feel great! I can't imagine it not being healthy for you, keep the foods fresh and be creative when you cook."

Or how about Chef Karen Larkin who makes soups from scratch every morning at her McKinleyville, California café: "I love this diet! It really works! I add a few different herbs and spices to each batch to give it an international twist. For example, I add chopped cilantro, a little chili powder, and cumin to give it a Southwestern flavor; some oregano, basil, and fresh garlic for an Italian taste; a little curry powder mixed into the cooking soup and chopped fresh mint leaves for garnish on top when serving to give it a unique Moroccan flavor; shrimp or fish bullion, a little soy sauce, and some fresh bean sprouts, minus the tomatoes for an exotic Oriental sensation; chanterelle mushrooms and a pinch of thyme and rosemary minus the tomatoes for a wonderful French taste. All very yummy!"

Natalie from Nixa, Missouri, says: I have used this soup many times, and lose about 10 pounds each week! My family likes it too, so I add ground turkey or diced Chicken to it and we have a meal! It is a great way to clean out your system and make you feel great, if followed correctly! I use it for a week, off a week, on a week, and off a week, and usually can keep the weight off for a year or 2, if I am careful! Just be sure to take your vitamins, and eat all the stuff it calls for.

Laurie W. from Berks, UK, says: "You cannot fail to lose weight on this diet (as long as you don't cheat!). I lost 8-lbs the first time, and then on my second go 5 weeks later, I lost another 7lbs! Providing you don't stuff yourself silly on the first day off the diet, then eat sensibly, there is no reason why you should put the weight back on! Good luck."

Lenia Kallis from Nicosia, Cyprus, says: "Cutting the cabbage into big chunks makes you feel fuller as you are eating something solid. And yes it tastes great and you still lose the weight. On the fruit day I make a nice big fruit salad with a little orange juice and consume it the whole day. On the vegetable day I sauté the vegetables in a non stick pan and add a little soy sauce to fool myself I am eating Chinese food. I use Thousand Island dressing for the baked potato. Yes I too lost 9 pounds on it. And it is not that difficult either with the above recommendations. It is imperative that you have one good multivitamin a day, plus a half to one teaspoon of water soluble vitamin C three times a day. It really helps the energy levels. All the above make the diet easier to follow and the results are dramatic. It motivates me also to go on a better and more nutritional diet the week after. I feel that it is good for me as I do not consume any meats for the first 4 days of the diet. Good luck to all."

– CHAPTER THIRTY EIGHT –

ADD TO YOUR BODY

Water
Drink 7 to 8 glasses of pure water daily.

Why? It helps keep your blood flowing, your brain cells floating, flushes out toxins and helps keep all organs and joints lubricated.

Exercise
Get at least one-half hour of exercise daily.

Why? It helps keep your body flexible and youthful, helps stabilize your weight and keeps good circulation for sustained energy. Enjoy stretching, walking, jogging, yoga, biking and use weight-bearing exercises to keep your bones strong and your muscles toned. (A simple formula that works: Walk as fast as you can as far as you can.)

Fruits
Eat all kinds and all colors of fruits – fresh or frozen.

Why? These most natural of foods for your body help keep you in alkaline/acid balance and potassium balance, and provide cleansing fiber, vitamins and minerals. They are delicious and beautiful, and wonderful in smoothies, too!

Vegetables

Eat plenty of fresh or frozen vegetables, especially dark green leafy and colorful vegetables.

Why? They help keep your eyesight sharp, are high in fiber, high in vitamins and minerals, including the calcium your body can use. Enjoy fresh vegetable juices!

Whole Grains

Eat wheat, oats, ground flaxseed, brown rice, etc.

Why? They are excellent sources of fiber, vital B-vitamins (found in the bran and germ), protein and minerals. Satisfying fiber in plant protein helps to keep your daily intake of protein between 45-50 grams for better calcium balance from the vegetables.

Nuts and Seeds

Eat plenty of flaxseed, walnuts, pecans, almonds, sunflower seeds, pumpkin seeds, etc.

Why? They are excellent sources of essential fatty acids like Omega-3, vegetable protein, fiber, vitamins, and minerals that keep your heart healthy and help control blood sugar. Fresh nuts and seeds mixed with a little dried fruit make a satisfying snack. Sprout the seeds to add enrichment to salads.

Legumes
Consume beans, peas and lentils.

Why? They provide your body with essential nutrients, good plant protein and high fiber, which help prevent the buildup of toxins and heavy metals (such as lead). Legumes give long-term energy and satisfy your hunger.

Good Fat
Use extra virgin olive oil, flax oil, canola oil, sunflower oil, avocados and cold-water fish such as tuna, salmon and sardines.

Why? Your body needs good fat that provides essential fatty acids such as Omega-3 to keep your skin, hair, and eyes glowing. Good fats also help keep your joints and organs operating smoothly. They should make up about 15-20 percent of your daily calories. Did you know that 60 percent of brain tissue is composed of essential fatty acids and your brain suffers if you don't eat good fatty acids?

NOTE: If you have blood sugar problems (high or low) – eat small amounts of the above foods five to six times daily. Your body can properly digest smaller amounts of food and will be able to use all of it for energy. When your blood sugar drops, you will have a tendency to overeat and/or crave sweets.

– CHAPTER THIRTY NINE –

REMOVE FROM YOUR BODY

Sugar

Why? Refined sugar starts out as a food, but it is refined down to just the sweetness with no fiber or nutrients to slow its entry into your blood stream. When your pancreas tries to limit the amount of sugar getting to your brain, it thinks the sugar will continue coming into your body at the same rate, so too much is turned into glycogen and stored as fat. This leaves your body in the state of "low blood sugar." Low blood sugar can trigger anxiety, irritability, sluggishness, headaches, depression, etc. and can lead to diabetes.

Artificial sweetener, color and flavoring

Why? These substances increase your desire for sweets and bad fats by 300 percent. If you doubt this, go off your "diet soda" for a week or so and then have some and find out how hungry you get. Artificial sweeteners have been found inside brain tumors . . . which just could be the result of your body trying to get it out of your blood stream. Artificial flavoring is a cover for appetite stimulants to cause you to over eat. Artificial colors contribute to attention and behavior problems.

Caffeinated Beverages

Gradually cut out or significantly reduce the intake of coffee, Coke, Pepsi, Mountain Dew and other caffeinated drinks.

Why? Because they have a dehydrating effect and large amounts can cause jitters, irritability, insomnia, and elevated blood pressure. If you want something hot, try hot water with fresh lemon – delicious. Scientific studies have found that drinking even five glasses of water daily can cut the chance of heart disease by 50 percent. However, it has also been shown that just five eight-ounce servings of *other* drinks can *increase* your chance of heart disease by 257 percent. Harvard studies have found that 1 can of soda a day increase the chances of diabetes by 83% for a 9-year-old child! (Unfortunately, many children consume five or more 12-ounce cans of soda daily!)

Partially Hydrogenated Fat

Eliminate these bad fats that are found in most margarines, snack foods and many of the processed foods we eat.

Why? These fats are high in trans fat, which scientific studies show is a big contributor to heart disease, cancer and obesity. With the over-consumption of calories, diabetes has increased over 900 percent in the last 15 years. They are in all fast foods. Read the labels!

Foods made with Refined, Enriched White Flour

Why? This flour quickly turns into glucose in the blood stream and, when coupled with sugar, lactose and caffeine, your body will quickly undergo severe stress. This combination can also contribute to the loss of B-vitamins and other vital nutrients.

Excessive Amounts of Animal Products

Why? These foods lack fiber, and you should consume no more than three ounces of animal products two or three times weekly for best health.

Cigarettes

Why? They have an even higher correlation with cancer and heart disease than formerly thought. For natural help and a high rate of success to cease smoking seek the assistance of Acupuncture and/or hypnosis coupled with high intake of Vitamin C and B complex vitamins with your good diet and exercise.

Alcohol

Why? Alcoholic beverages can cause mood swings and rapid fluctuations in your blood sugar. In excess, they can lead to addiction, emotional problems, gastritis, ulcers, pancreatitis, hepatitis, cirrhosis, hypoglycemia, diabetes, gout and nerve and brain dysfunction. A little wine occasionally doesn't seem to be a problem, but freshly juiced red and purple grape juices are even better for your overall health. (If you have never had freshly juiced fruit or vegetables - obtaining a good juicer would be a wonderful addition to your household.)

– CHAPTER FORTY –

THE 20 BEST, HEALTHIEST FAT-BURNING FOODS

Apples: A rich source of soluble fiber – with no sodium, saturated fat or cholesterol. Apples gently raise your blood sugar level, prevent hunger pains, and keep you fuller, longer.

Barley: This grain is high in fiber and low in fat. Studies at the University of Wisconsin indicate that is can lower cholesterol by up to 15 percent – and it contains powerful anti-cancer agents.

Berries: Berries have fiber to satisfy your hunger, and natural fructose sugar to satisfy your sweet tooth. They are also a great source of potassium, which can help control blood pressure. Blueberries are particularly healthful.

Broccoli: This is the number-one cancer preventing vegetable. It is high in fiber and has no fat. Plus, it has loads of beta-carotene, 21 times the RDA for vitamin C – and it's an excellent source of calcium.

Buckwheat: Research has shown that buckwheat helps regulate blood sugar and lower cholesterol levels.

Cabbage: Excellent protection against colon cancer. In fact, surveys in the U.S, Greece and Japan have shown that people who eat lots of cabbage have the lowest incidences of colon cancer – and the lowest death rates.

Garlic: Cooked or raw, garlic stimulates the immune system, reduces the risk of cancer, and even helps normalize blood pressure.

Grapefruit: Like all citrus fruits, grapefruit is high in vitamin C and potassium, and virtually free of fat and sodium. It is also high in pectin, the fiber that has been linked to lowering the bad fat.

Greens: Collard greens, kale, Swiss chard, turnip greens, beet greens, chicory and spinach are full of fiber and free of fat. They supply plenty of filling bulk along with iron, beta carotene, and vitamins A, C and E.

Hot Peppers: Rich in vitamins A and C, calcium, phosphorus, iron and magnesium, high in fiber, fat free, low in sodium – and they speed up metabolism and great for good circulation when taken in capsule form.

Kiwi: High in vitamin C and potassium – and delicious.

Legumes: Peas, kidney beans, lentils, chick peas, and other legumes have the most protein with the least amount of fat of any food. Plus, they are high in potassium, low in sodium – and contain powerful anti-cancer agents.

Melons: Melons have the highest fiber content of just about any food plus lots of vitamins A and C, and potassium.

Mustard: Temporarily speeds up the metabolism by as much as 20 to 25 percent for several hours. That makes it possible for you to burn an extra 45 calories for every 700 calories you eat.

Oats and oat bran: This whole grain is a great source of fiber that helps lower bad cholesterol (by as much as 20 percent), and regulate blood sugar. It's a proven weight loss aid. In one study, subjects lost 3 pounds in two months simply by adding 6 or 7 tablespoons of oat bran to their daily diets. (Paul's Oats by Natural Ovens Bakery is a delicious source of oat fiber.)

Onions: Yellow onions, red onions, scallions, leeks – all onions can add years to your life. They lower the bad cholesterol, thin your blood, and help protect against high blood pressure and heart disease.

Tofu: A 2-1/2 inch square of this low-fat meat substitute supplies a hefty nine grams of protein. It also supplies calcium and iron, with almost no sodium and no saturated fat. It speeds up your metabolism, lowers cholesterol, and protects against cancer.

Tomatoes: Low in fat and sodium, high in potassium, and rich in fiber, tomatoes are one of the most versatile ingredients in any cook's repertoire.

Whole-grain breads: Pumpernickel, whole-wheat, multi-grain, and oatmeal breads are a natural source of fiber and complex carbohydrates – and protein.

This list was generated from Delicious Foods that Make you LOSE WEIGHT by Robert D. Willix, Jr., M.D.

A FINAL NOTE

We hope you have enjoyed "*Keeping It Off*" and truly hope it can help you get rid of pounds you want to lose and then to be able to keep them off.
If you would like more information about Natural Ovens Bakery products or any of the information presented in this booklet, please call 800-558-3535 and ask to speak with Melissa.